ATHENE Series

General Editors

Gloria Bowles
Renate Klein
Janice Raymond

Consulting Editor

Dale Spender

The Athene Series assumes that all those who are concerned with formulating explanations of the way the world works need to know and appreciate the significance of basic feminist principles.

The growth of feminist research internationally has called into question almost all aspects of social organization in our culture. The Athene Series focuses on the construction of knowledge and the exclusion of women from the process—both as theorists and subjects of study—and offers innovative studies that challenge established theories and research.

ATHENE, the Olympian goddess of wisdom, was honored by the ancient Greeks as the patron of arts and sciences and guardian of cities. She represented both peace and the intellectual aspect of war. Her mother, Metis, was a Titan and presided over all knowledge. While pregnant with Athene, Metis was swallowed whole by Zeus. Some say this was his attempt to embody her supreme wisdom. The original Athene is thus twice born: once of her strong mother, Metis, and once more out of the head of Zeus. According to feminist myth, there is a "third birth" of Athene when she stops being an agent and mouthpiece of Zeus and male dominance, and returns to her original source: the wisdom of womankind.

Surviving the Dalkon Shield IUD

WOMEN v. The Pharmaceutical Industry

KAREN M. HICKS

FOREWORD BY
Diana Scully

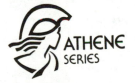
ATHENE
SERIES

TEACHERS COLLEGE PRESS
Teachers College, Columbia University
New York and London

Published by Teachers College Press, 1234 Amsterdam Avenue
New York, New York

Library of Congress Cataloging-in-Publication Data

Hicks, Karen M., 1947–
    Surviving the Dalkon shield IUD : women v. the pharmaceutical
industry / Karen M. Hicks.
        p.   cm. — (Athene series)
    Includes bibliographical references and index,
    ISBN 0-8077-6271-7 (cloth : acid-free paper). — ISBN
0-8077-6270-9 (paper : acid-free paper)
    1. A.H. Robins Company. 2. Dalkon Shield (Intrauterine
contraceptive) 3. Intrauterine contraceptives—Complications.
II. Series.
HD9995.C64A2344   1993
338.7'616139435—dc20   93-36105

    ISBN 0-8077-6270-9 (pa.)
    ISBN 0-8077-6271-7 (cl.)

Printed on acid-free paper
Manufactured in the United States of America
99 98 97 96 95 94 93   8 7 6 5 4 3 2 1

Contents

Foreword

I met Karen Hicks, founder of the Dalkon Shield Information Network (DSIN), on her first trip to Richmond, Virginia, in May 1987. Richmond is the home of the A. H. Robins Co., the pharmaceutical house that invented and manufactured the Dalkon Shield intrauterine device. Karen contacted me because she had read my book, *Men Who Control Women's Health*, and thought I might be an ally in the Dalkon Shield claimants' cause. I clearly recall the day Karen sat in my university office and told me about her dread of coming to Richmond because of all it symbolized for her, about the suffering she had experienced as a result of the Dalkon Shield, and about her insecurity over the enormous task she was about to undertake. I encouraged her to go forward but also warned that she would never again be the same: It would be a transforming experience. I was right!

Surviving the Dalkon Shield IUD is Karen Hicks's compelling account of the Dalkon Shield tragedy and how a small group of women took on the corporate giant, A. H. Robins. It is also a story of corporate greed and callous disregard for the reproductive health and emotional well-being of women told by a survivor of the Dalkon Shield. In promoting and selling the Dalkon Shield, despite knowledge of its defective design utilizing a string that promoted infection, A. H. Robins caused countless numbers of women severe side effects that included bleeding, pain, inflamed and perforated uteri, spontaneous abortions, infertility, sterility, birth defects in offspring, and even, in some cases, death.

There is another side to the Dalkon Shield story. It stimulated a highly effective and passionate grassroots organization, DSIN, and changed the lives of many of the women who struggled to force A. H. Robins to take responsibility for its actions and compensate victims for their suffering and loss. There were major frustrations along the way, too: As candidly recounted by Karen Hicks, long and draining litigation, A. H. Robins's bankruptcy tactics, the lack of support for DSIN among some feminist organizations, and internal disagreements among DSIN leaders all took a toll on DSIN members. Richmond, if not hostile, was less than welcoming. In fact, at the height of Robins's bankruptcy proceeding, local DJs frequently aired a song that lamented the possibility of lost jobs for Robins's workers and complained about the "selfishness" of Dalkon Shield claimants! Even among local feminists there was apathy for the claimants' cause. Indeed, the 1976 Virginia celebration of the United Nations Decade of Women was held at the Robins Center, a costly athletic facility given by the Robins family to the University of Richmond. Few saw the irony of holding a celebration of women in a facility built, no doubt at least in part, with Dalkon Shield profits.

Yet amidst the frustration and tragedy there was empowerment. I recall the Richmond rally during one of the first Dalkon Shield proceedings. The woman walking beside me, obviously tired and upset, had received a notice of the proceeding from the court. Debilitated by her Dalkon Shield-related injuries and believing that her claim would be settled that day, she used her life savings to fly from New York to Richmond. The cab ride from the airport the day before had taken her last dollar and, with no money for food, she had slept in the park that night. Now she had learned that there would be no settlement that day or any time soon. Yet, as I drove her to the airport that night, she told me she didn't regret her decision to come to Richmond. For her, being with other survivors and participating in the rally restored her sense of personal control and elevated her spirits.

Clearly, through DSIN, members experienced the personal as political and learned that through collective action, women can make a difference. Credit for that goes to Karen Hicks, who undoubtedly knows that empowering women is the best feminist work. *Surviving the Dalkon Shield IUD* is an important chapter in our herstory.

Diana Scully
Richmond, Virginia

Acknowledgements

My sincerest gratitude goes to the Dalkon Shield women who collaborated with me on this book: Sherry Fletcher, Jan Thompson, Shirley Nichols, Fran Cleary, Joanne Ackerman, Gloria Manago, Victoria Pratt, Rita Lauderdale, Cinders Murdock-Vaughan, and Donna Reeck. Thanks also to Dalkon Shield women and men who shared themselves: Constance Miller, Katie Falls, Audrey Konstans, Russell and Mary Stone, and Deirdre Hill-Brown. I am also grateful to Deb Oliver for her many talents in preparing the manuscript and to Mark Howells for his assistance. And finally, my love and appreciation to Barry Bean, my partner in life, who never wavered from encouraging me under the strains of also living this story twice—first in the making of it and now in the telling.

1 The Context of the Injustice

More than 2 million U.S. women and a total of 4 million women worldwide used the Dalkon Shield intrauterine birth control device (IUD) between 1970 and 1974. The Shield was promoted as the "Cadillac of contraception." For three years while the Shield was being prescribed, neither physicians nor women were warned of the dangers it posed as a defective birth control product. Because it was distributed on a mass scale, the Dalkon Shield is now acknowledged as the most notorious contraceptive, one that caused widespread and extensive damages to its users.

The Dalkon Shield became a major women's health care tragedy, one that was caused by corporate misconduct on the part of Dr. Hugh Davis, the Shield's inventor, and corporate executives of A. H. Robins Company, the pharmaceutical firm that began to manufacture the device in the early 1970s. This threat to women's bodies was exacerbated by the failure of the Food and Drug Administration (FDA) to act: It neither demanded the removal of the Shield from the market nor instituted a comprehensive recall of this defective product.

The history of the Shield's development, marketing, and distribution, as well as the complex and lengthy litigation surrounding Robins, has been ably documented (Mintz, 1985; Perry & Dawson, 1985; Sobol, 1991). Among the many people who place the blame for this disaster on the profit motive is U.S. District Court Judge Miles Lord, who presided over some 23 Shield-related lawsuits in 1984. In his courtroom, Lord chastised Robins executives for not warning women and their doctors about the Shield's dangers:

> The only conceivable reasons you have not recalled this product are that it would hurt your balance sheet and alert women who already have been harmed that you may be liable for their injuries. You have taken the bottom line as your guiding beacon, and the low road as your route. This is corporate irresponsibility at its meanest. (Mintz, 1985, p. 267)

The extensively documented Dalkon Shield injuries now on record include severe hemorrhaging, septic abortions, infected miscarriages, an epidemic of pelvic inflammatory disease (PID) among users, ectopic pregnancies, perforated uteri, infertility, mutilated and lost reproductive organs, birth defects in children, and at least 20 documented deaths. The psychosocial damages include emotional trauma from infertility and loss of bodily integrity, economic hardship due to lost income or career opportunities, and strained or failed personal relationships.

Thousands of women continue to suffer from injuries that originally were unexplained and often were untreated or misdiagnosed because vital information was suppressed for so many years. Although the litigation surrounding this case has inspired countless newspaper articles and several books, very little has been made public about the specific adverse effects this tragedy has had on the hundreds of thousands of injured women and their significant others.

The victims of cases involving the reckless endangerment of the public health are typically submerged in a culture of silence to the extent that they themselves hardly know the true reasons for their physical maladies; thus they do not understand the connections between those injuries and the resulting array of problems they face. Corporations like Robins have the power and privilege to engage in tactics of protracted denial and cover-up, which have the consequence of delaying early medical treatments and increasing the prospects of chronic and life-threatening damage. Therefore the full scope of the injustice can remain misunderstood and underappreciated for decades, making the social reform of medicine difficult or impossible.

This book examines the embryonic stage of a social movement initiated by a small group of former Dalkon Shield users who became enraged by their circumstances, striking out of isolation and powerlessness to battle the official worldview of them and to propose an agenda for social reform in medical and pharmaceutical practice. The Dalkon Shield users who became members and leaders of the Dalkon Shield Information Network (DSIN) are the subjects of this book. The political activism of the women who formed DSIN was partially a response to their rage about their shared stories of medical horror. These women interrupted the culture of silence and gave voice to the injustice they had lived with for the better part of 20 years.

Because I am the principal founder of the DSIN, its story is, in large measure, my own story. As a Dalkon Shield survivor and a social scientist, I am in a unique position to document the history of this instance of women organizing for social change. I have worked, essentially, in two modes as a researcher: first as an interested party, a participant seeking useful information about the legal process, and then, after largely withdrawing after three years of direct participation, as a social scientist analyzing the process. The insider's perspective of a social movement in progress is, to my knowledge, almost nonexistent in scholarly studies of social movements. My intent is to document the mobilization impulses that led to political activism, the strategies that emerged to challenge the powerful institutions, the complex web of relations, and the transformation of some "ordinary" women into battleworthy warriors.

A more thorough understanding of the women injured by the Dalkon Shield, as well as of the range of negative physical, psychological, and socioeconomic sequelae, would reveal how deeply pernicious victimization of health care consumers, particularly women, is and how it is perpetuated by two powerful social institutions—medicine and the law. Individuals who remain isolated from one another as private clients of doctors, therapists, or lawyers are unable to establish the links necessary to fight for just solutions to cases of medical abuse. Documenting the commonalities of experience is a necessary step in focusing on the structural conditions that tolerate this type of medical exploitation of and violence against women. Fine (1986) argues that research on such collective experience is urgently needed in order to draw cases that maintain pervasive victim-blaming ideologies, such as the Dalkon Shield case, into the public consciousness. Only then can programs of reform be formulated.

MEDICAL FRAUD PUTS WOMEN AT RISK

Intrauterine birth control devices are an ancient form of contraception. There are historical references to herders in desert cultures placing stones in the uteri of camels during long, arduous treks across rugged terrain. The first attempts to introduce IUDs into widespread human use during the late 1800s failed because so many women died of massive infections.

Most modern IUDs are made of polyethylene, and many medicated models contain copper or hormones. They require sophisticated physician/clinician skill for insertion and removal as well as for patient management during use. IUDs are inserted into the uterus via the vagina. The cervix (which connects the vagina to the uterus) must be stretched with a special instrument during insertion and removal. Most IUD models have tailstrings attached, which hang down into the vagina and are used to check for proper placement and for removal. The medical literature is inconclusive on the precise mechanism of

IUD action. The IUD may prevent fertilization of the egg (if it contains copper or hormones), but, more often, it interferes with implantation of an embryo. Therefore it can be categorized both as a contraceptive and as a contragestive device.

The development of modern antibiotics in the early 1900s made IUDs feasible, and the "pill scare" in the late 1960s led to an era of intense competition among pharmaceutical companies to find a profitable alternative to the early oral contraceptive, which had caused serious injury. In 1973, Dr. Joseph Mamana, the chief of the FDA's Medical Devices Compliance Section, was quoted in a newspaper interview:

> Anyone—it doesn't even have to be a doctor—can go down to his basement, get a few hairpins, stick them together, and call it an IUD. There's nothing we can do about it until someone is injured or dies. ("Interview . . . ," 1973, p. 16)

The Dalkon Shield IUD was A. H. Robins's first plunge into gynecological/reproductive products. For the previous hundred years of its existence, this family-owned and -operated pharmaceutical company had built a strong, positive reputation on cold and flu remedies. Robins's aggressive marketing campaign and advertising literature claimed that the Dalkon Shield was "the superior" birth control method, with *no* systemic bodily harm or ill effects. These claims turned out to be not only patently false but life-threatening to the women who entrusted their family-planning needs to this product. In the early weeks of the Shield's mass distribution, physicians began sending in alarming reports of injury to Robins's medical staff; yet company executives embarked on a strategy of deliberately and willfully suppressing the vital information that could have prevented the coming mass tragedy (Mintz, 1985).

The leading theory about how the Dalkon Shield causes injury cites a phenomenon called *wicking*, involving the multifilament tailstring, that hangs downward from the uterus into the vagina. All previous IUD models had monofilament tailstrings. The grooves in the twisted filaments, which were tied into a double knot on the Shield, allowed bacteria to settle there and ultimately to travel up into the sterile uterus. Wayne Crowder, a quality control supervisor at the Robins's manufacturing plant, observed problems with the strings and speculated about the dangers of infection and septic abortion. He recommended methods to correct the problems, but company officials ignored him. When he persisted in his demands, for reasons of conscience, he was fired: Julian Ross, his supervisor at the plant, told him his conscience did not pay his salary (Mintz, 1985, p. 141).

The transcripts of a 1973 congressional hearing and Robins's company records that were part of a federal grand jury investigation reveal the magnitude of the corporate and medical misconduct. The 1973 hearing, conducted by the U.S. House of Representatives, was precipitated by the Dalkon Shield crisis. Pressure for the hearing came from doctors and women's health activists alarmed by the proliferation of severe and life-threatening injuries to Dalkon Shield users. The congressional hearing was necessary before the FDA would regulate IUDs.

The documents from the congressional hearing and the federal investigation reveal a scientific fraud with far-reaching consequences. Dr. Hugh Davis, professor of obstetrics and gynecology and head of a gynecologic clinic at Johns Hopkins University, co-invented the Shield with Irwin Lerner, an inventor and electrical engineer. Davis falsified his original experimental data, had his research published in a prestigious medical journal, and then lied under oath about his personal financial stake in the manufacture and sale of the device (Mintz, 1985). In 1970, Davis sold the Shield's distribution rights to the A. H. Robins Company, which rushed the Shield into production in order to capitalize on the birth control pill scare.

The Dalkon Shield studies were dangerously defective. Only Dr. Davis conducted the brief (12 months) and severely flawed research. He counted his 640 subjects as a grand total of 3,549 woman-months of experience, but this figure was grossly misleading, since the average user in his study used the Shield for only five months (Mintz, 1985, p. 31). Davis recommended that these women use a back-up method of birth control in the first three months post-insertion (Perry & Dawson, 1985). Additionally, his study had a 60% discontinuation rate. Because Davis used the established "life-table" method (the benchmark protocol used in contraceptive trials), the women who dropped out of the clinical trials were lost to follow-up, so complications were not included in the study's results (Committee on Government Operations, p. 61). Clearly, data about the women who discontinued use during the trials would have been invaluable.

Davis wrote a laudatory article on the Dalkon Shield, which was published in the *American Journal of Obstetrics and Gynecology* (Davis, 1970). He claimed both a superior low-pregnancy and low-complication rate for the Shield relative to other IUDs then on the market. Davis's study slipped through the system unchecked: No physician appears to have examined the validity of his study before its publication. Davis himself never conducted a safety study, never identified himself as co-inventor of the Shield, and never mentioned his recommendation of a back-up method. His article was misrepresented "as the work of an unbiased, scientific observer" (Perry & Dawson, 1985, p. 35).

Davis actually submitted the draft of his article only days after the study was completed, which meant that his pregnancy statistics did not reflect women who might have become pregnant in the latter part of the study. In fact, that is exactly what happened. The actual pregnancy rate was between 3% and 5%, which proved the Dalkon Shield to be decidedly inferior to both the pill and other IUDs on the market (Perry & Dawson, 1985). By 1971, the Dalkon Shield had become the most popular IUD on the market, primarily because of the favorable reception of Davis's published article.

A. H. ROBINS SHIELDS ITS ASSETS

Following a series of lawsuits between 1978 and 1984, the A. H. Robins Company petitioned the U.S. Bankruptcy Court in 1985 for protection under Chapter 11 of the U.S. Bankruptcy Code. Chapter 11 requires a distressed business to formulate a plan of reorganization in order to satisfy all its debtors. At the time of the Robins petition, the company was financially robust, with cash on hand and virtually no corporate debt. The company claimed, however, that the escalating number of Dalkon Shield lawsuits would jeopardize its solvency. This petition for protection from bankruptcy coincided with a growing number of monetary damage awards to women in state courts around the country.

Although the initial injuries occurred in the early 1970s, most women did not discover that the Dalkon Shield was the actual cause of their physical damages until around 1986, as a result of the publicity surrounding these bankruptcy proceedings. The bankruptcy court ordered Robins in 1985 to implement a publicity campaign to notify injured parties of their rights to file claims for damages. More than 327,000 women filed injury claims against Robins in bankruptcy court by the court-imposed deadline of April 1986. However, court-imposed protocol reduced that original number to approximately 197,000 legitimate claims.

This decade-long delay in public acknowledgment of possible liability exacerbated the early injuries and left thousands of women at grave risk for developing serious, even life-threatening, disease. Even throughout the bankruptcy proceedings, A. H. Robins Company spokespersons continued to assert that "the product is pure" (Morris, 1988c). They implied, as they had in the earlier lawsuits, that the alleged sexual lifestyles of women (promiscuity and poor hygiene) caused the physical injuries.

In 1988, the sale of the A. H. Robins Company to American Home Products (AHP), a pharmaceutical giant, emerged as the bankruptcy court's solution to the litigation. In February 1988, the reorganization plan was submitted to the bankruptcy court, presided over by U.S. District Court Judge Robert R. Merhige, Jr. By July, Robins's stockholders and a vast majority of the nearly 200,000 women, men, and children whose claims had survived several of the previous court-imposed protocols and deadlines voted on and overwhelmingly approved the plan. By becoming "claimants" against the company, these people surrendered their legal rights to pursue individual lawsuits against Robins, Aetna (Robins's insurer), their doctors, or any other potentially liable entities.[1] The Dalkon Shield Claimants Trust (referred to herein as "the Trust") was infused by $2.45 billion in cash in December 1989, the official date of the plan's consummation. The creation of the Trust was a contentious and heated process during the bankruptcy proceedings, involving the pharmaceutical and insurance industries, court officials, and plaintiffs' attorneys.

In spite of the dazzling size of the Trust, most of the claimants will receive what they and many experienced personal-injury lawyers consider inadequate compensation. As of July 1992, approximately 137,000 of the 197,000 claims have been settled. Of these, 115,000 women received settlements of $1,000 or less. Other women have received various amounts ranging from $1,000 to more than $150,000. A few "baby cases" (children born with birth defects) are reportedly worth about $1 million each. Due to the secrecy of the Trust's operations and the lack of access to information imposed by the Trust officials on almost all facets of the Trust's operation, only Trust officials have specific information about the process used to determine the settlements.

Several new legal precedents were established during Robins's Chapter 11 litigation, including (1) allowing immediate reimbursement to stockholders at the time of the sale, contrary to the existing Bankruptcy Code, which specifies that stockholder payments are to be made only *after* all outstanding debts are settled, (2) giving immunity to third parties not under bankruptcy law protection, in this case the Aetna Insurance Company,[2] and (3) assigning greatly increased authority to the judge sitting on this case[3] in managing the Trust. Indeed, Judge Merhige has been the subject of criticism over his handling of the case and the Trust (Labaton, 1988a, 1988b; Mintz, 1986a, 1986b, 1989b, 1989c; Sobol, 1991).

SILENCING THE VICTIMS

In the Dalkon Shield case, an essentially private source of suffering and injustice, with a private and intimate meaning based on women's sexuality and reproduction, was compounded by a deliberate and cynical pattern of control and manipulation of information that in fact contributed to a secondary victimization of these women. The unwavering public posture of denial from A. H. Robins—which insisted that its product was pure—and the corporation's amply documented complicity in deception and cover-up of its direct role together demand that women's reality about the initial and subsequent victimization be publicized and validated.

The silencing of victims is demonstrated by the repeated use of two mechanisms of information control and manipulation that put the victims at a disadvantage relative to the corporate, medical, and legal interests in this case: (1) denial of wrongdoing on the part of A. H. Robins officials, as already mentioned, and (2) withholding of vital information necessary for the women to receive just treatment and the fullest guarantee of their legal rights. This pattern of withholding vital information by everyone—first by the inventor, then by the A. H. Robins Company and the courts, and now by the Dalkon Shield Claimants Trust—compounded the problems these women have faced for decades. Women were also managed behind closed doors by a varying group of experts, such as doctors, therapists, and lawyers. They had little, if any, opportunity to discover that so many other women had had similar experiences. The victims, as a collective, were socially invisible until the grass-roots activism began in 1987 during the Robins bankruptcy proceedings. The early letters and phone calls to DSIN speak to this effect. The following letter sent to DSIN is typical of thousands of women's responses:

> It has been 16½ years since my Dalkon Shield was removed along with all my reproductive organs and until now, I have felt so totally alone in my agony. Until I read your comments in *The Wall Street Journal*, my emotional, physical, and legal problems seemed insurmountable. (Letter #306)

During the early phase of the bankruptcy proceedings in Richmond, public perception surrounding the case was shaped by the carefully constructed press statements from high-status officials in Robins's public relations department and from the court. The impression created in the media was that Robins was bankrupt, which was far from the truth. And during the first two years of its Chapter 11 petition in the bankruptcy court, the presiding judge granted Robins six extensions on the submission of a reorganization plan, further delaying the process. As some women experienced it, this was business as usual for Robins, with injured women hanging in limbo indefinitely.

The inadequacy of the court-imposed campaign to locate users was dramatized by the unexpected deluge of telephone calls from women who read an April 1989 issue of *Women's World*, a supermarket tabloid, which ran a story on the Shield and listed DSIN's telephone number ("Are You a Victim . . . ," 1989). More than 500 women called the DSIN hotline over the next several weeks. Most of the women calling claimed that this was the very first piece of information they had ever seen about the dangers of the Dalkon Shield. A preliminary analysis of those telephone call records revealed that women were calling from virtually every state in the United States.

Other anecdotes continue to indicate the lack of resolution to this tragedy. In July 1992, the DSIN hotline received a call from a woman who was still wearing the Shield. She was experiencing traumatic reproductive health problems, and an x-ray had revealed the device. She had been told years ago that it had fallen out.

CORPORATE, MEDICAL, AND LEGAL INTERESTS

According to Petchesky (1984), the real power base that defines women's contraceptive choices resides in the juncture of medical, corporate, and legal interests. Throughout the series of events detailed in this book, I expand Petchesky's hypothesis to include the notion that the consequences of contraceptive tragedy are also defined by the same triad of power. An analysis of the material basis of this case demonstrates that socioeconomic inequities, which favor corporate interests over the rights of injured parties, have prevailed. The sizable assets of the errant corporation have been kept in the hands of A. H. Robins officials and other economic elites, in the following ways:

1. In 1987 alone, Robins's total disbursements for the bankruptcy litigation exceeded $13 million, with payments going to 16 law firms, 6 accounting firms, and 13 court-appointed professional consultants ("Professional Fees," 1988). In 1988, Robins paid $25 million to Rorer, another large pharmaceutical company, as a merger termination fee for reneging on its agreement. (Several companies had

courted Robins, but AHP won the bidding war.) By contrast, not one Dalkon Shield claimant received a penny of financial compensation for life-threatening injuries or urgently needed medical treatments until the bankruptcy litigation was completed at the end of 1989. More than 35,000 claimants are still awaiting review of their claims as of 1992.

2. The value of A. H. Robins shareholders' stock increased fourfold as a result of the merger deal. The Robins family and corporate officials, who owned 42% of A. H. Robins stock, exchanged their shares in Robins for AHP stock. In this transaction, Robins family members and executives, taken in the aggregate, became the largest shareholder of AHP. Additionally, AHP received sizable tax breaks for buying a so-called distressed company.

3. The Robins Company and family successfully separated a substantial portion of total assets and net worth from the Chapter 11 proceeding because many of Robins's subsidiaries were not included in the Chapter 11 proceeding. Furthermore, the Robins family owns other valuable enterprises, including several telecommunications businesses and a wine import business. In 1992, Dalkon Shield women and attorneys were shocked to learn about the election of E. C. Robins, Jr., to the post of honorary president of the American Pharmaceutical Association (M. Pretl, personal communication, February 18, 1992).

4. The Chapter 11 reorganization plan granted the corporation, the Robins family, and all other third parties (primarily the Aetna Surety and Casualty Company) permanent and total immunity from any further Dalkon Shield–related civil litigation. Therefore Dalkon Shield injured parties can turn nowhere else for financial settlements if the Trust is inadequate to provide compensation for their injuries.

5. The Trust has a 20-year lifespan, and its administrative costs have been estimated variously at between 10% and 25% of the total funds. Every important sector of the Trust's operation utilizes services in Richmond, Virginia, Robins's hometown—including the bank that handles the accounts; the real estate leased to house the claims facility; the legal counsel representing the Trust; trade services such as printers, computers, and so forth; and the more than 200 employees, who were recruited principally from the Richmond area.

6. If women hire attorneys, they will pay contingency fees. Many of the lawyers are charging standard contingency fees (roughly one-third) or higher, plus expenses, in spite of the fact that the case

preparation to the Trust is straightforward and simple in comparison with pursuing of an individual lawsuit and going to trial. One DSIN leader was awarded a $127,000 settlement by the Trust in 1992; after her lawyer subtracted his fees, she was left with $84,000.

It is the view of many Dalkon Shield users and all the DSIN leaders that the financial compensation program resulting from the Robins bankruptcy settlement does not represent social justice. Their concept of social justice involves three themes. First, DSIN sought to have a major health agency sponsor and conduct a comprehensive, worldwide product recall of the Dalkon Shield. Second, the leaders demanded an investigation of the FDA and its mishandling of the regulatory process. Strengthening the FDA is seen as necessary for the protection of future populations of women and other medical consumers. Third, DSIN was passionate in its desire to see criminal charges brought against the inventor and corporate officials in Robins and Aetna who were responsible for this tragedy. In spite of repeated pleas by DSIN leaders and other public interest groups throughout a three-year period, the Justice Department dropped its criminal investigation within one month of the Robins–American Home Products merger (Geyelin, 1990).

THE BOOK

The task of this book is twofold: The first task is to document the continuing victimization of and injustice to Dalkon Shield users during the years 1986–1990, during which corporate interests took precedence over human welfare. The second task is to describe and analyze the educational and political strategies of a small group of Dalkon Shield women who challenged the legal system and presented their own definition of social justice for this population of women and medical consumers.

This book provides a rare perspective in the literature on social movements in two ways. First, this case study covers the formative period of the movement. Most studies of social movements take place after the movement is over and stress the end, not the beginning. This book can add valuable data on the ideas, tactics, personalities, alliances, and decisions that contributed to the successes and limitations of this instance of women organizing for medical reform. Second, as a former Dalkon Shield user and founder of DSIN, I offer an insider's perspective on the mechanisms of oppression, the nature of the

injustice as it is viewed and interpreted by the victims, and the transformation of women from the status of socially invisible and powerless victims to that of empowered survivors. The central themes in
this book include the psychological and philosophical roots of activism, the conditions under which activism became necessary, and the
particular issues that consumed the leaders of this organization. The
outcome of the analysis is a model curriculum of empowerment
applicable to other cases and circumstances of victimization.

DSIN members transformed the private trauma into a public
agenda of social reform. Their activism asserted the victims' perspective and challenged the dominant worldview of events, particularly
about the legal solution. Their rage upon gathering and learning the
true cause of their personal health misfortunes led them to thrust
themselves into a legal process that neither asked for nor wanted their
participation. The women presented the contradictions and discrep-
ancies in experience reported by those in high- and low-power positions (Kidder & Fine, 1986). The women in DSIN have also publicly
articulated the negative human consequences of high-tech contraceptive methods, challenging the population control movement's enthusiasm for widespread distribution of IUDs and other high-tech methods of birth control that alter a woman's body, either chemically
(through synthetic sex hormones) or biologically (through implanted
devices).

Records of victimization and models of empowerment are an
essential contribution to our understanding resolutions to social problems of exploitation and people's attempts to challenge the status quo.
"When previously private problems become visible, social scientists
and activists must expose ideologies such as 'they must have asked
for it' that justify inequitable social arrangements" (Kidder & Fine,
1986, p. 57).

The Structure and Method of the Book

Chapter 2 reviews the medical literature on contraceptive development
and IUDs and describes specific experiences of women worldwide. It
details the misogyny and patriarchial control of contraception that
subjects women to this form of medical violence. Chapter 3 provides
the chronology of events in the life history of DSIN, spanning a three-
year period. The complexity and urgency of developing relationships
to other organizations and other Dalkon Shield women is treated in
Chapter 4. Chapter 5 presents an analysis of the strengths and limitations of this social movement. The final chapter provides a model,

or curriculum of empowerment, and suggests other investigations that are still urgently needed in order for us to understand the comprehensive impact of this case.

The research for this book was praxis-oriented; that is, the research applied a critical and empowering model of inquiry and action for building a more just society (Lather, 1986). In my original mode as a woman struggling to understand what had happened to me, I searched continually for data. I was driven to know and understand what was going on in the long, drawn-out bankruptcy proceeding involving A. H. Robins because I had suffered a life-threatening injury as a direct result of using its product. These considerations also affected many thousands of other injured women, entwining our lives in that litigation. My intense personal stake in obtaining information plunged me into tedious searches of court records, many trips to Richmond, endless telephone conversations with women and lawyers, and direct, ongoing, daily contact with many of the principal legal parties to the case. This continued for the better part of a three-year period.

In my determination to make sense out of the process I was engaged in, I kept detailed notes of every telephone conversation as well as a voice-tape diary. In no other way would I have been able to gather the enormous quantity of data now in my possession.

As I came to appreciate the complexity of this case, I decided to keep track of all the people, places, and events that I participated in, believing that a detailed, written record would ensure that I could accurately reconstruct and interpret information given to me and that it would generally aid the process of informing other women of the case's progress. In short, all data collection has been systematic and structured from the beginning of my participation, even though the original goal was not research, but action.

I used the following data collection techniques:

- Handwritten notes (duly dated and timed) of virtually every telephone conversation I have had with Dalkon Shield survivors, many lawyers who are principal parties to the case, court officials, allied organizations, and numerous national press people with whom I have had continous contact
- The voice-tape diary I started keeping on almost a daily basis for a two-year period (now entirely transcribed into more than 200 pages), which stands as my field notes
- Newspaper clipping files, organized by month, of most national news stories that appeared during the Chapter 11 negotiations

- Voluminous files of related newspaper and law journal articles, magazine interviews, and analyses
- Videotapes of DSIN events, television news stories, and interviews with survivors, recorded by DSIN and other women around the country
- Court documents and briefs related to the estimation-of-claims process and most other court events during 1988
- More than 400 unsolicited letters received from Dalkon Shield survivors who wrote to DSIN and volunteered parts of their stories
- Correspondence and other documents generated by other Dalkon Shield survivors working on special projects
- All correspondence between DSIN and other Dalkon Shield groups, allied organizations, the court, and plaintiffs' lawyers
- All press releases, press statements, news reports, and speeches produced by DSIN during its period of greatest activity between July 1987 and December 1988, including 12 major public press- and court-related events.

SUMMARY

The Dalkon Shield tragedy has far-reaching consequences for women's reproductive health care, contraceptive development and distribution, and the legal rights of people injured by products known to be defective or dangerous. In the case of the Dalkon Shield, young and healthy women at the height of their childbearing potential were exposed to life-threatening and sterility-producing iatrogenic illness. Any disease or illness resulting from medical intervention or treatment is iatrogenic: The development of disease is an unintended outcome arising either from medical error or from unknown risks of a medical procedure or medication.

This story of Dalkon Shield women who became part of a grassroots organization called the Dalkon Shield Information Network (DSIN) and who publicly delineated the catastrophic results of a particular form of contraception on their lives may help to promote reform in women's reproductive health care, contraceptive development protocols, and medico-pharmaceutical practices.

2 Medical Violence Against Women

The analysis in this book utilizes a conflict-of-interests perspective (Kidder & Fine, 1986) to explain medical violence against women. This perspective involves a structural analysis of a collective problem and the action of people to fight against an agent of injustice—in the present case, the multinational pharmaceutical industry. The conflict-of-interest approach engenders alternative explanations of events, reaching beyond the elites who generally control the flow of information and the interpretation of events.

By medical violence, I mean all needless operations, misdiagnoses, and failed medical interventions performed on victims with less social power than medical professionals. Medical violence reflects and reinforces patriarchal values and social structures. It also results in an enormous profit to the medical elites and in great cost, both physical and financial, to the victims.

CORPORATE MISCONDUCT IMPERILS HUMAN WELFARE

The link between corporate and medical misbehavior and social injustice is receiving increased attention in the literature. Mokhiber (1989) has published *Corporate Crime and Violence*, a compendium of 36 cases of corporate abuses of the public trust, including the Dalkon Shield case. His profiles are confined to a superficial background description of U.S. corporations that have engaged in deliberate and ruthless behavior, including intricate cover-ups and strategies of denial. Although some of these cases are not of medical origin, they nonetheless present life-threatening consequences for persons exposed to the dangers. Mokhiber, writing from the legal perspective and proposing remediation in both the civil and criminal justice systems, does not detail victim responses, but he acknowledges that such data are vital to aid future efforts to gain justice.

Gerry Spence, attorney and author of *With Justice for None* (1989), describes U.S. business patterns of exploitation as well as abuses within the legal system, and he also proposes reforms in the civil justice system.

Chellis Glendinning, a woman injured by both the birth control pill and the Dalkon Shield, has written a book titled *When Technology Wounds* (1990). She cites the commonalities among the many and growing instances of mass disasters from chemical and reproductive technology, not exclusively the province of women's suffering. Her book focuses on the personal healing process that is essential in order for individuals to reconcile their victimization.

THE LEGACY OF MEDICAL SEXISM

Real social change directed at improving medical care for women can be facilitated by examining and redressing the social and economic arrangements that keep women sick and powerless relative to the elites who perpetuate and benefit from the system. Through its power and privilege, the A. H. Robins Company maintained for years the misconception that women's injuries from the Dalkon Shield were caused by promiscuity and poor personal hygiene, thereby shifting attention away from themselves and perpetuating a "blame-the-victim" posture. This tactic delayed important medical diagnoses and treatments that might have partially rectified the early damages.

This book focuses on the medical specialty of gynecology and reproductive medicine, with its pervasive tendency to discount the serious risks of medically invasive drugs and devices prescribed to women who use the health care system for quality-of-life needs, not for illness. The history of gynecologic medicine is replete with examples of medically induced (iatrogenic) illness in otherwise healthy women. Those cases include the vaginal adenocarcinomas of daughters born to women who were prescribed DES during pregnancy, the birth defects associated with pregnant women's use of the drug thalidomide, the cardiovascular and circulatory problems experienced by women who used the early birth control pill, unnecessary gynecologic surgery, including clitorectomy and hysterectomy, and silicone breast implants, to name a few.[1] The unethical medico-pharmaceutical behaviors involved in the Dalkon Shield circumstance created a needless iatrogenic disaster on a massive scale. When such injuries occur, a formerly healthy person may suffer permanent damage, require lifetime medical care, or even die as the consequence of agreeing to a medical procedure designed to enhance her life.

Contemporary feminist historians demonstrate that, prior to the early twentieth century, U.S. women's reproductive healthcare was attended to within a female culture that offered sympathetic personal support and guidance (Smith-Rosenberg, 1973; Smith-Rosenberg & Rosenberg, 1973). In the 1800s, women tended to the reproductive needs, including abortion, of other women as autonomous midwives and general healers. As medical knowledge grew, traditional medicine evolved as an almost exclusively white, male profession. Beginning in 1910, licensing laws enacted throughout the United States created a medical monopoly over obstetrical and gynecological care, and midwifery was outlawed (Ehrenreich & English, 1973). That midwifery was outlawed undermined and diminished women's culture, and women became medically dependent on men for nonpathological health matters such as birthing and birth control (Millett, 1970).

The injuries suffered by Dalkon Shield users remained misdiagnosed and mistreated for the better part of 20 years. Scores of women who contacted DSIN reported that they had been diagnosed neurotic at some point during these years. The catch-all diagnosis of the "neurotic woman" is the prime means by which some doctors delegitimate and mistreat true illnesses, neutralize women's power, and keep women in a passive status relative to physicians. Ruzek (1978) articulates:

> Medical sexism is especially pernicious for it is veiled in the medical mystique of science and rationality. Because women have been largely excluded from acquiring scientific knowledge, they have had little opportunity to question medical practices. Thus, their complaints have been disregarded as emotionalism or neuroticism. (p. 12)

THE WOMEN'S HEALTH MOVEMENT

From its beginning in the late 1960s as an outgrowth of the women's rights movement, the women's health movement has provided a sociocultural explanation for the dehumanization and exploitation of women in the health care system, which has intensified since the control of women's health shifted from midwives to gynecologists. Feminist health activists assailed the hegemonic medical model as the principal means of affirming patriarchal control over women's lives, particularly through the high status, prestige, and power accorded to the reproductive medical specialty of obstetrics and gynecology (OB/GYN). Many feminists see this medical specialty as a devastating form of sexual politics that puts the interests of men ahead of women's health and makes physicians the social control agents of women (Ruzek, 1978).

The unrestrained autonomy that Dr. Hugh Davis enjoyed during his research and development on the Dalkon Shield in the 1960s is a familiar theme in the history of gynecology and women's reproductive medicine. J. Marion Sims, an Alabama physician who has been called "the father of gynecology," "perfected" gynecologic surgeries in the 1850s. His subjects were slave women, "a readily available source of material for surgical experimentation" (Scully, 1980, p. 42). Without anesthesia, he performed repeated surgical experiments on these women—whose owners gave him permission to do so. By the time of his death, he was heralded as "the evangelist of healing to women" (p. 46). Other early gynecologists of the late nineteenth century are revered in parallel terms.

Diana Scully's (1980, in press) study of medical schools and the current training of obstetricians and gynecologists, which are dominated and controlled by male physicians and professors, lays bare the continuing exploitive traditions in this women's health specialty. OB/GYN residents are socialized into a culture of medical/surgical abuse against women, not very different from that of Sims. Poor, minority women in large teaching hospitals fare the worst, as residents scramble to get enough surgical practice.

Vicente Navarro (1976) asserted the patriarchal nature of medicine by using the metaphor of the family. Physicians dominate at the top layer, as the symbolic fathers—the decision makers and power figures. Nurses and other paraprofessionals are the symbolic mothers; and patients are the symbolic children, whose needs are the object of the father's and mother's concern. Navarro reveals the sweeping potential for profound inequities within this hierarchical system, created by a pervasive ideology of sexism, racism, and class discrimination.

Within the entire range of health and body issues that fall under the umbrella of the women's health movement, I find few written records of women's personal experiences of organizing to fight against specific medical abuses. The history of the Boston Women's Health Book Collective represents the development of a feminist-inspired group organized around these general themes of exploitation and abuse. Social critics have written about the injustice involved in cases such as those involving thalidomide, the early birth control pill, DES, and the Dalkon Shield, but scant records detail women's organizing efforts around their personal experiences of health and body abuses, such as caesarean and hysterectomy prevention, the abuse of amniocentesis for gender preselection, DES daughters, and so forth. Written accounts of women's organizing attempts on specific health issues may accelerate and enhance the development of an ideology that will propel the social reform of medicine and women's health care.

SEXISM IN CONTRACEPTIVE RESEARCH

Hartmann (1987) has identified three biases in contraceptive development: (1) The contraceptive world is sexist—leaders and researchers are predominantly male, and female methods are their overwhelming focus; (2) the preference is for systemic and surgical methods, which receive 70% of all funds available for development, as opposed to barrier methods, which receive 2.2% of funds; and (3) greater concern is shown for efficacy than for safety, as less than 10% of total expenditures for contraceptive development since 1965 have been devoted to safety.

One chilling affirmation of the social context and medical sexism embedded in contraceptive development and use is the opening statement of Dr. J. Robert Willson at the First International Conference on Intra-Uterine Contraception, sponsored by the Population Council in 1962:

> They [IUDs] are horrible things, they produce infection, they are outmoded and not worth using . . . but suppose one does develop an intrauterine infection and suppose she does end up with a hysterectomy and bilateral salpingo-oophorectomy? How serious is that for the particular patient and for the population of the world in general? Not very. . . . Perhaps the individual patient is expendable in the general scheme of things, particularly if the infection she acquires is sterilizing but not lethal. (Tietze & Lewitt, 1962, p. 3)

A hero in the history of Dalkon Shield litigation from the perspective of the former users is Miles Lord, a now-retired federal judge in Minnesota who presided over 21 Shield cases in 1984. In a bold move for which he was later censured by his peers, Judge Lord summoned Robins's executives into his courtroom and soundly chastised them for their misconduct. Part of his memorable speech dramatizes the sexism implicated in this specific contraceptive disaster:

> I dread to think what would have been the consequences if your victims had been men rather than women, women who seem through some

strange quirk of our society's mores to be expected to suffer pain, shame
and humiliation. (Perry & Dawson, 1985, p. 208)

Three books that present a comprehensive analysis of birth control politics in America all speak to the medical sexism embedded
within it. Gordon (1977), Petchesky (1984), and Hartmann (1987)
consider the economic, political, racial, and class factors that determine women's relation to medicine and family-planning distribution
systems. Gordon reviews the social history of birth control in America,
arguing that access to contraception has always been a matter of social
and political acceptability rather than of medicine and technology.
Petchesky and Hartmann argue that in reproductive health care, class
and race are the crucial determinants of women's risk of exposure to
involuntary sterilization, dangerous contraceptive drugs, and other
potentially harmful medical practices, such as unnecessary hysterectomy.

Birth Control Versus Population Control

Both Petchesky and Hartmann draw the critical distinction between
birth control and population control. Birth control involves an individual woman making personal decisions about a range of contraceptive methods. Population control, on the other hand, is the control
by authorities or elites over population size and composition, control that extends to sexuality, the physical health of women, the terms
and conditions of motherhood, and the structure of the family.
    Hartmann proposes that the population control establishment is
totally preoccupied with fast and effective contraceptive methods, to
the neglect of health and safety issues. She criticizes the International
Planned Parenthood Federation (IPPF) for marrying itself to population control and thus divorcing itself from the concern for women's
health and well-being. She also details the U.S. government's complicity abroad through the population policies of the United States
Agency for International Development (USAID). Foreign aid has been
tied to the adoption of the population control agenda orchestrated
within the United States and executed by IPPF clinics around the globe.
USAID bought the surplus Dalkon Shield IUDs and distributed some of
them through IPPF clinics overseas after they were removed from the
U.S. market (Ehrenreich, Dowie, & Minkin, 1979).
    During the 1973 congressional hearings on IUDs, doctors who tes-
tified pointed out that many of the modern IUD inventors were closely
affiliated with the population control movement. Jack Lippes, inven-

tor of the Lippes Loop IUD, was the medical director of Planned Parenthood and World Population. Howard Tatum, inventor of various
IUDs, including the copper-bearing models, worked for the Population
Council. Dr. Alan Guttmacher, part of the population control movement, allowed testing of the first modern IUD in his clinic. In addition to his faculty appointment in the OB/GYN department at Johns
Hopkins, Hugh Davis was Associate Professor of International Health,
Population, and Family Health. Christopher Tietze (1967), a high-profile population scientist at the Population Council in New York City,
developed modern contraceptive research protocols and methods. He
is characterized as a "zealous advocate of IUDs" in an annotated bib-
liography on IUDs compiled by Dr. Russel Thomsen, a physician who
testified at the congressional hearings (Committee on Government
Operations, 1973, p. 71).

Hartmann uses the term *fervor* to describe the work rate of experts
developing high-tech contraceptives, namely synthetic hormones and
IUDs. The population control and family-planning editors of The
biennial series *Contraceptive Technology* admit to an extensive bias
among clinicians in favor of the pill and IUD. "In spite of their safety,
condoms, diaphragms, and foam get a very 'bad press' within many
family planning clinics and offices" (Hatcher et al., 1986, p. 103).

Hartmann and Petchesky both expose the paradoxical fact that
the safer barrier methods are more likely to give women true reproductive control, yet these methods are denigrated and ignored, even
by Planned Parenthood, the champion of legal abortion and every
woman's right to reproductive control. Hartmann argues that the
thrust of contraceptive research today is, in fact, an attempt to remove
contraception control from women.

A woman's birth control options are crucially different depending on her socioeconomic class and race. Petchesky refutes the notion
that women have individual *choice* and argues that fertility control is
not a personal, private matter, but rather that it occurs within defi-
nite social contexts and sexual power relations. The link between the
population control community's goal of zero population growth (ZPG)
in the late 1960s and the decisions women made about adopting the
Dalkon Shield underscores this point. Many Dalkon Shield women
recall the ZPG rhetoric clearly as they recount their decisions to use
the device. The choices, therefore, are more dependent on social and
material conditions in the larger societal context. Petchesky asserts
that "The 'right to choose' means very little when women are powerless to determine the social framework that conditions their options"
(Petchesky, 1984, p. 11).

Trivializing the Side Effects

Both Petchesky and Hartmann reviewed statistics on contraceptive outcome and found that physical damage or injury is the greatest single obstacle to the use of family-planning services as well as the major reason for discontinuing contraception. The World Bank's *World Development Report 1984* confirms this trend. One survey in the Philippines revealed that 66% of women stopped using the pill and 43% the IUD for reasons related directly to physical injury (World Bank, 1984). Petchesky (1984) also confirms the declining use of the pill and the IUD from the 1960s to the 1970s, with two-thirds of women in every age and racial group dropping out due to "experienced physical problems" (p. 186).

Adverse side effects of and high discontinuation rates for high-tech contraceptive methods are not adequately acknowledged or used to redirect contraceptive research and policy. Testimony from medical experts at the 1973 congressional hearings assailed the misuse of the *life-table method* for compiling and reporting experimental data on IUD use. This statistical method had been devised in the early 1960s by the Population Council's Dr. Christopher Tietze. Tietze advocated the exclusion of all patients lost to follow-up in IUD trials. This rate varied from 13% to 30% (Committee on Government Operations, 1973, p. 10). He rationalized this statistical method for use with so-called fluid populations, where new subjects are added and old ones drop out. This method was applied to the only Dalkon Shield study conducted by Hugh Davis.

Dr. Russel Thomsen, a witness at the 1973 hearings, pointed out that study protocols on IUDs were not controlled, experimental designs that tracked a well-defined subject population, but were instead based on a situation in which women using the device actually and unknowingly become the study population. Therefore information on complications among former users was neither collected nor reported. Thomsen commented on these IUD guidelines:

> This "life table method" of statistical evaluation has been blatantly misused as a method of predicting effectiveness or side effects of IUDs. Actual rates are usually eventually shown to be much different than those which were predicted and then used as the basis of advertising claims. (Committee on Government Operations, 1973, p. 72)

Dr. Hugh Davis was director of family-planning services at Johns Hopkins University Hospital, and the product development and earliest trials of the Dalkon Shield took place in his public clinic, where most of his patients were poor. The earliest Dalkon Shield models thus were tried out on Davis's patients. He simply inserted various models into poor, mostly African-American, women from Baltimore's inner city. They were the original guinea pigs (Mintz, 1985). The women did not sign consent forms, and it is not known what they were even told. Davis apparently enjoyed total autonomy; it is not clear what kind of accountability the hospital required of him.

Katie Falls, an African-American woman and Dalkon Shield survivor who became editor of the DSIN newsletter, wrote cynically about women's victimization, having been victimized herself. The following is excerpted from an article she wrote that appeared in the DSIN newsletter:

> We have the *right* to submit our bodies to an altered state of reproduction. We have the *right* to make our reproductive choices, according to information supplied by the manufacturer, approved by the FDA and prescribed by a medical professional. . . . Should a tragedy occur as a result of the contraceptive method we have chosen, WE HAVE THE RIGHT TO REMAIN SILENT! (Falls, 1989, p. 3)

The margin for abuse is great in a system in which doctors enjoy almost unlimited autonomy while developing medically invasive devices. Their word alone should not suffice as "evidence" of safety and efficacy, but doctors are extended an extensive privilege of belief from a trusting public. This is one of the reasons that the Dalkon Shield exploded into popularity. Barbara Seaman, a women's health activist and co-founder of the National Women's Health Network, was researching and writing *The Doctors' Case Against the Pill* (1969) around the time that Davis was experimenting with the Shield. She interviewed Davis for her book and wrote very positively about the Dalkon Shield, quoting his claims for its superiority. Davis ultimately wrote the foreword, titled "A Public Scandal," to her book. Ironically, he expressed outrage at the lack of disclosure about the problems associated with the birth control pill and took this opportunity to glorify the Dalkon Shield as the most effective and *safest* form of contraception.

Dr. Russel Thomsen testified at the 1973 hearings that dire complications among his Dalkon Shield patients led him to conduct his own research into IUDs. He found evidence that, despite adequate proof that IUDs are capable of producing serious and even fatal complications, they are "in that lucrative arena of medical devices which breeds poor research, deceptive advertising, and actual medical hucksterism" (Committee on Government Operations, 1973, p. 50).

An intensive literature search on all types of IUDs reveals plenty of evidence to warrant a more restrained and less fervent approach to the mass adoption of this contraceptive technology, particularly in environments that are not equipped to deal with the negative outcomes. Acker's study (1973) showed that 29 out of 87 women had significant electrocardiogram changes while undergoing IUD insertions. In a review of 18 case-control IUD studies, Keith and Berger (1984) found that 12 showed a positive relationship between IUDs and PID. They also noted that the incidence of a formerly uncommon condition called *pelvic actinomycosis* soared after the adoption of IUDs. The same report showed a sixfold higher rate of ectopic pregnancy and a fourfold higher rate of chronic pelvic pain among IUD users. A news brief in the May 1987 issue of *Contraceptive Technology Update* ("IUDs May Promote Infection . . . ") discussed the research of three microbiologists who speculated, based on their laboratory experiments, that IUD design and the use of copper may cause infections. Kirshon and Poindexter (1988) found a significantly higher incidence of endometriosis in former IUD users, which they hypothesized could be due to a retrograde flow of prolific menses, which is characteristic among IUD users.

Several studies also allude to the serious underreporting of the incidence of infections and other damage because statistics are based only on women requiring hospitalization (Burkman, 1981). Several doctors testifying at the 1973 congressional hearing also speculated about the possibility of underreporting due to doctors' fears about medicolegal liability. The problem is compounded by the number of different specialists women are likely to seek out for wellness care and sickness care:

> A Planned Parenthood clinic can simply concern itself with the expense of inserting 1,000 IUDs versus keeping 1,000 women on the pill. But that same clinic rarely sees its own major IUD-related complications, let alone foots the bill for the treatment of those complications. (Committee on Government Operations, 1973, p. 57)

Generally, potential IUD damages were widely understood before the Dalkon Shield was marketed. Sheldon Segal, a career scientist with the Population Council, wrote during the 1960s about the damage to endometrial tissue exposed to IUDs. Segal's (1968) report on the biological action of IUDs graphically decribed damaging ulcerations in the uterine endometrial lining adjacent to IUD placement. He acknowledged that microscopic analyses of the endometrial lining directly adjacent to the device revealed the lining to be thin and ulcerated.

He also described chronic endometritis (inflammation of the endo-metrium).

Since Segal's early reports, population control and other scientists are still reporting pelvic infections and other damages among IUD users more than 20 years later. Although an advocate of IUDs, Dr. Howard Tatum is nevertheless convinced of a connection between tailed IUDs and uterine infection. In 1986, he was refining the development of tailless, magnetic IUDs, which would be removed with an electronic retriever ("Despite Liability . . . ," 1986).

Dr. John G. Madry, Jr., one of the first physicians to testify at the 1973 congressional hearings, recounted his frustration when trying to acquire information on adverse IUD outcomes. He was motivated to pursue information because of injuries he had observed in more than 20 patients he had fitted with IUDs. He contacted 12 different organizations but was not able to locate any statistics. Because he was alarmed and troubled by the dissonance between the lack of answers on injury and the high praise for IUDs by government and the population control establishment, he made a personal decision to stop inserting IUDs:

> It became more apparent that the technical truth regarding IUD-related morbidity and mortality lay somewhere behind the adversary assertions of fact as presented by IUD advocates, who excluded uncertainties and minimized complications in their reports. (Committee on Government Operations, 1973, p. 5)

In spite of these troubling questions, the Population Council continues to champion IUDs. In a 1987 press release, the World Health Organization (WHO) cited the conclusions of "a scientific group of experts" (not named) who met at WHO and gave IUDs a "clean bill of health" ("WHO Gives IUDs . . . ," 1987). In 1989, the ParaGard Copper T 380A IUD was introduced to the market. *Glamour* magazine featured the new IUD positively in an article, asserting that "the IUD is back—with a clean bill of health" (Young, 1989, p. 60).

THE DALKON SHIELD AS WAR ON THE WOMB

Women's Stories

The discounting of women's experience with the Dalkon Shield is repeated endlessly in the stories of women who contacted the DSIN. That women's real complaints about the device have been trivialized is consistent with Martin's analysis of science's mechanistic approach to women's reproductive functions. She has documented the cultural assumptions at the foundation of medical practice in the United States.

> Many elements of modern medical science have been held to contribute to a fragmentation of the unity of the person. When science treats the person as a machine and assumes the body can be fixed by mechanical manipulations, it ignores, and it encourages us to ignore, other aspects of ourselves, such as our emotions or our relations to other people. Recent technological developments have allowed this tendency to progress very far. (Martin, 1987, p. 19)

Martin offers a penetrating analysis of the medico-scientific constructs of women's bodies and reproductive functions in *The Woman in the Body* (1987), along with a perspective on the sets of cultural metaphors, medical metaphors, and imagery associated with the uterus, menstruation, and pregnancy. She elaborates on the scientific construction of the uterus in economic terms—as a machine of (re)production. The cultural negativism toward menstruation is coupled with the "failure" of the uterus to produce.

I would expand on her concept of the uterus as machine by looking also at the medico-scientific construction of pregnancy prevention. The summarizing statement of a research report on the evaluation of IUDs conducted by the American Medical Association and published in the *Journal of the American Medical Association* states: "The IUDs and the oral contraceptives represent another of *man's* successful efforts toward intelligent *control of his environment*" [emphasis added] ("Evaluation of . . . ," 1967, p. 647).

The rhetoric of IUD advocates is reminiscent not of the economy, but of war, and more specifically, of weaponry and war machinery. Jack Freund, a Robins employee summoned to testify in the 1973 congressional hearing, called the Dalkon Shield "a valuable part of the physician's contraceptive *armamentarium*" [emphasis added] (Committee on Government Operations, 1973, p. 305). Dr. Louise Tyrer, a witness at the same hearings, referred also to the IUD's place in the contraceptive *armamentarium* (p. 366). The uterus is all too often made into a battleground on which outside forces—anti-abortion fanatics, population control zealots—attempt to subvert women's individual control of their bodies by restricting access to fertility-related healthcare and information.

The image of weaponry is also evoked in the description of the electronic retriever device to be used with Tatum's tailless, magnetic

IUDs that appeared in a journal targeted to population control and family-planning experts.

> Tatum and his collaborators invented a special retrieval device—shaped like a pistol with a long, thin barrel attached to a hand grip. At the tip of the barrel are tiny "grasping hands" that can be extended, opened, and closed by squeezing the hand grip. The barrel tip also contains magnetic sensors, enabling the clinician to use the retriever "like a video game," commented Tatum. ("Despite Liability . . . ," 1986, p. 142).

In 1984 Judge Miles Lord, mentioned previously, referred to Dalkon Shields as "instruments of death, of mutilation, of disease" and continued the warfare metaphor when he spoke of the countless women who still carried a "deadly depth charge in their wombs, ready to explode at any time" (Perry & Dawson, 1985, p. 208).

Mary Stone, an early member of DSIN, was Hugh Davis's patient during his early trials of the device. She recalled those days in an interview in the *Village Voice* (Eagan, 1988). Mary was 18 years old when a friend recommended Davis to her in the early 1970s. Although she developed pain and heavy bleeding immediately after he inserted the Dalkon Shield, he dismissed her complaints, asserting that this was "normal." A few months later, she insisted on removal, and "to his amazement, [it] was bent out of shape by the force of her uterine cramps" (Eagan, p. 24). He immediately inserted another. Her problems persisted, but Davis was unsympathetic. Her experience over a period of years is chilling. Never once did he call her by her real name; he only referred to her as "Suzi Q." Stone now describes Davis as "arrogant, rude, abrupt" (Eagan, p. 24). She struggles to contain her anger when she recalls the living horror she endured and the man responsible for it:

> In December 1973, she was in his office again for a checkup. "He started screaming at me," she recalls. "'You pulled it out!'" he accused. "How could I pull it out?" she asks rhetorically. "That thing had *teeth*!" Unable to locate the second Shield, Davis inserted a third.
> "That's when I really started having pain. I'd bleed for 14 days, 18 days. And I had this pain in my side. At one visit, he pointed to my head, and said 'That's where your pain is!' In August 1975, I finally insisted on having it out. He was furious. He tore it out of me and threw it in the trash can." (Eagan, p. 24)

Eventually Davis did exploratory surgery, which showed scarring on Mary's fallopian tubes, evidence of pelvic infection. He prescribed antibiotics and warm douches. For many years, she believed her problems were all her own fault. She finally consulted another doctor in 1977. Almost immediately, he performed a total hysterectomy, leaving her sterilized. Mary was 25 years old. During the surgery, this doctor discovered the second Dalkon Shield embedded in the wall of her uterus. To this day, she suffers unrelenting pelvic pain related to these injuries. She is often unable to work.

Fran Cleary, the DSIN chapter leader in Richmond, has an astonishing personal story, one which reveals depths of horror. (See Appendix A for a complete transcript of the interview for this book.) In the 1970s, Fran's father-in-law was Robert Nickless, then vice-president of international marketing for the Dalkon Shield. Nickless (now deceased) apparently knew enough about the Shield to have written an early memo (in 1970) in which he raised the question of the Shield's wicking problem to other Robins's officials (Perry & Dawson, 1985).

Soon after he wrote this memo, Nickless sang only the highest praises for the Dalkon Shield and coaxed Cleary into having one inserted. Both Cleary, a biologist, and her husband were skeptical about the Shield, and they questioned Nickless in great detail about side effects and safety. Cleary eventually agreed to use the Shield, but within weeks after insertion, she was hospitalized with a life-threatening pelvic infection. She endured years of pain, infertility problems, and aggressive surgeries. She did not discover the extent of her father-in-law's complicity until she joined DSIN in 1988 and read Mintz's (1985) book, which was mailed out to new members.

Since then, Cleary has struggled to understand what transpired between the time Nickless expressed early skepticism and his conversion to being a champion of the device. Nickless was the Robins official who traveled extensively throughout Asia, promoting the Dalkon Shield in many countries (Ehrenreich et al., 1979). He never told Cleary what he knew about the Shield, nor did he ever discuss the true etiology of her injury with her. There were times when he lied outright to both his son and his daughter-in-law, as Cleary describes:

> It soured me, and I'm bitter about it, and I've become more bitter about a lot of things as a consequence, and that's not good but that's the way it is. The fact that I was lied to for so many years by someone I loved, and who loved me, and that money and success meant more than the truth, and after I found this out, I saw it again and again in the courts, when the Robins

Company was continually trying to use the women who were injured and make them look like the guilty parties, when all along they knew they were the guilty parties, and they continued to do that all along, and they're still doing it right up to this day.

Women who have written or spoken out as part of their activism in DSIN invoke the imagery of violence, which they perceive from being on the receiving end. Women repeatedly use terms such as *medical rape* and *medical holocaust*. Sybil Shainwald, women's health activist, attorney, and former board president of the National Women's Health Network, refers to case of the Dalkon Shield as the "Bhopal of the women's health movement." In the public speech I gave at the first Richmond protest march in 1987, I used the metaphor of "war on the womb" to characterize the Dalkon Shield injustice. The women in the Los Angeles chapter of DSIN wore red and black clothing, symbolizing blood and death, to every organized meeting they held.

Katie Falls, DSIN member and newsletter editor in 1989, also made the analogy of Dalkon Shield users to casualties of war. She describes herself in a handmade pamphlet she created in 1990 titled "Dalkon Shield Brigade: POWs of the Civil War, 1960–1980":

> ABOUT THE AUTHOR: She was inducted into the Dalkon Shield brigade, in late 1973. This unit held the front lines for the Women's Liberation and Black Power movements. Their main objectives were to do their patriotic best to reach Population 0, by the year 2000. Many women joined the brigade, in their desire to do their part. The author was one which [sic] did not escape the draft. (personal communication, 1990)

Imagery: Flying Uteri and Magic Crabs

The imagery of women used in the slick ads developed by the Robins advertising staff during the heyday of the Dalkon Shield's distribution is profoundly degrading. Three particularly offensive advertisements ran in all the leading OB/GYN journals and other medical journals in the early 1970s. The most bizarre advertisement showed a uterus floating in space in the foreground, as if it were approaching the reader (see Figure 2.1). Inside the uterine cavity, a Dalkon Shield appears to rest comfortably. This surreal depiction is reminiscent of the objectification of women's bodies—an internal objectification in this case. What could a uterus without a woman surrounding it mean to the men who conceived this advertising campaign?

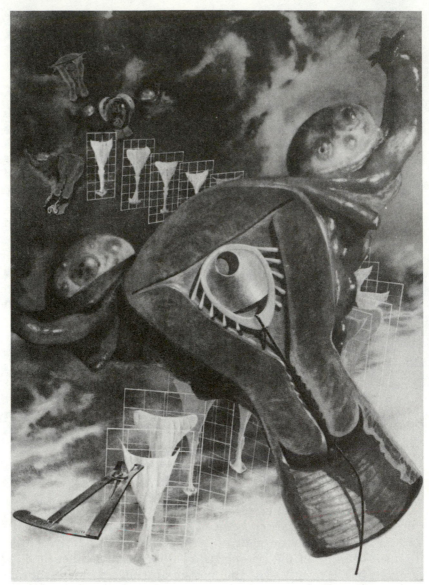

FIGURE 2.1 This advertisement, which appeared in various medical journals in 1970 and 1971, was dubbed "The Flying Uterus" by plaintiffs
attorneys.

The caption proudly asserts that the Dalkon Shield is the "only IUD anatomically engineered for optimum uterine placement, fit, tolerance, and retention."

Other symbols in the background of the advertisement include what appears to be an engineering calibration tool, as well as other floating uteri, impaled on a backdrop of scientific chart grids. In a bit of macabre humor, plaintiffs' lawyers dubbed this infamous advertisement "the flying uterus." In hindsight, it is unbelievable that a rational person could look at that device and not question the danger those tailfins would pose to a uterus or a cervix. It is easy to imagine the fins constantly gouging and piercing the uterine wall, not resting quietly at all. Doctors and women were told that the common response of heavy bleeding was a "normal" side effect. Women now rephrase this bleeding as *hemorrhaging*.

Another advertisement vividly depicts one doctor's admiration for the device (see Figure 2.2). The doctor is gazing at the Dalkon Shield on its inserter stick in the palm of his hand. He appears to be in a hypnotic trance. What was the potential for cervical laceration during insertion or removal? Why were more questions not asked about the dangers posed by the Shield, the inserter stick, the insertion process itself, or any combination of the three?

The third advertisement identifies four types of women as ideal "candidates" for the Shield (see Figure 2.3). The "disorganized woman" cannot get anything done on schedule; the "clinic patient" is not sufficiently motivated to take the pill; the "pill reactor" cannot tolerate the troublesome side effects of oral contraceptives; and the "nullip" (never-pregnant woman), for whom Robins claimed a special, smaller Dalkon Shield was superior to every other IUD on the market.

In the course of contacting or joining DSIN, many women shared their ghastly, traumatic insertion and removal experiences. Cate Breslin (1989), a "nullip" freelance writer, dubbed this device "the magic crab" and wrote of her own insertion experience:

> The ripping, overwhelming pain-shock is recalled mostly as a peeling sensation on the back of my skull, as if a lightning bolt had vaulted from my crotch out through my head. My gynecologist—a contraceptive specialist and medical-school professor—said with evident self-satisfaction, "There, that went in very nicely." He sent me home with codeine-laced pain pills, "in case you have any discomfort over the next few days." (1989, p. 46)

Audrey Konstans, another woman who wrote to DSIN, removed the Shield herself, and as she pulled it out, "a piece of white meat

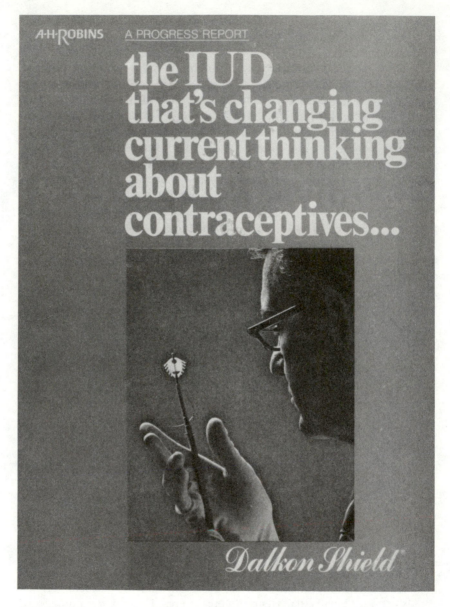

FIGURE 2.2 This advertisement also appeared in medical journals in 1971.

like chicken breast was hooked onto the Shield" (personal communication, 1987). There is no doubt that she is unknowingly referring
to a portion of her cervix. In a subsequent letter, she described this
trauma in verse:

> What is this thing inside of me? That hurts so terribly? Feels like
> a fire inside my womb. Could this object be my doom? Why
> didn't they tell me I would bleed and hurt? And with that
> thought, I gave a jerk. I sure hope I don't break this string. I just
> can't seem to rid me of this thing. My heart is pounding loudly
> in my ear. Why am I feeling so much fear? With another hard
> pull, another tug. Why what is this? It looks like a bug. And this
> strange looking thing has taken a bite out of me. There's pieces
> of my womb that I can see. (personal communication, 1988)

DOUBLE DANGER: SEXISM AND RACISM

Mistreatment of U.S. Women of Color

The Dalkon Shield presented an intensified risk to women of low
socioeconomic status who received poor-quality health care. Such
women who are injured by contraception are likely to suffer more
extensive and severe damage because of the marginal health care they
receive. The stories from women of color of lower socioeconomic
status—stories both of the injuries and of their mistreatment by the
medical system in the aftermath—are more hideous and gruesome than
the stories recounted by Caucasian, middle-class women. Countless
women of color received Dalkon Shields without their consent; doctors simply inserted them into their bodies without warning.

Sondra (pseudonym) is an African-American Catholic woman who
was abiding by her religion's ban on artificial birth control in 1973
and gave birth to a child when she was a 19-year-old college student.
She remembers the searing pain she felt during her first postpartum
exam: Her doctor had inserted a Dalkon Shield without even discussing it with her in advance. He told her that he was the one who knew
what was good for her.

In the ensuing months and years, the serious extent of her injuries and the lack of access to good-quality medical care combined to
cause her major distress. Sondra eventually lost custody of her son,
became homeless, and dissociated from reality during the pain and

Who are candidates for the Dalkon Shield?

The Nullip

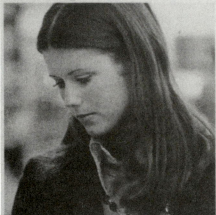

The "Pill Reactor"

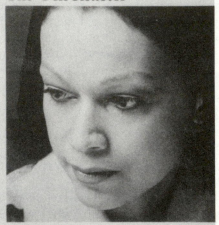

The applications of the Dalkon Shield are so universal that they cut across all socio-economic lines. They include all women who are not sufficiently motivated to take the Pill, ranging from the clinic patient* to the busy mother-career woman who has so many activities and interests that taking a pill simply slips her mind. They also include your patient who is so disorganized she can't seem to get anything done on schedule.

A prime candidate is the young nullip who will settle for nothing less than the most modern, trouble-free method of birth control. For her the Dalkon Shield is the logical IUD because it is also available in the smaller, nulliparous size. In fact, the Shield is the only IUD which has been anatomically engineered to fit the smaller uterine cavity of the nulliparous woman. Other IUD's have proved unsatisfactory because the patient cannot tolerate them. In addition to involuntary expulsions, severe cramping and bleeding have necessitated their removal for medical and personal reasons. Already more than 300,000 of the nulliparous size Shields have been sold.

Other candidates for the Shield include that large segment of women who cannot tolerate oral contraceptives, especially on a long-term basis because of the troublesome side effects. Some of these are patients whom you believe should

Nulliparous
model

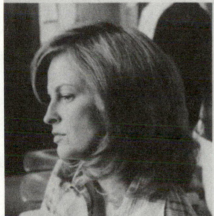
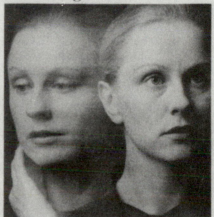

The"Clinic Patient"   The Disorganized Woman

be taken off the Pill; others may have asked you to substitute another method of birth control. Again, the Dalkon Shield is the contraceptive method of choice because it has no general effects on the body, blood, or brain. It cannot alter hormonal balance—cause depression, headache, weight gain, or fluid retention. Sustained menstrual irregularities are rare.

The modern woman also wants to be liberated from troublesome birth control devices such as the diaphragm. A few women can't use a diaphragm; many dislike the procedure of having to insert and remove it. Some may worry over whether or not it is in place. Not only is the Dalkon Shield a more effective contraceptive method than the diaphragm, condom, creams, foams, and jellies, but there is nothing to do before or after sexual relations. Neither partner is aware of its presence. In no way does it interfere with recommended feminine hygiene practices.

With the Dalkon Shield the patient can throw away her calendars, charts, and dispensers. No longer must she remember to take along her medication when she goes on a trip. She makes just one decision—to have the Dalkon Shield inserted. From this moment on, she is protected 24 hours a day.**

*Results of a study by Dr. Earl Siegel at North Carolina University School of Public Health show that women of a lower socio-economic status are more likely to continue with an IUD than with oral contraceptives. Of 351 women who originally accepted the Pill only 269 (55%) of 489 followed up were still using some form of contraception a year later. By contrast, of 131 women originally selecting an IUD, 100 of the 116 followed up (86%) were still contraceptors a year later.
Siegel, Earl, American Journal Public Health, 9:1886-98, 1971.

**A supplemental contraceptive method is recommended during a 2-3 month post-insertion adjustment phase.

FIGURE 2.3 This advertisement appeared in medical journals in 1971.

physical suffering she endured for more than a decade. She would often sleep on a beach at night, because there the gushing blood could drain into the ground. At other times, in desperate poverty, she cut up pieces of old shower curtains for sanitary pads.

Katie Falls, quoted previously, began to write as a therapeutic way of expressing her rage for her own mistreatment:

> I can only guess how many times I have wished that someone, anyone, would listen to what I have to say and read between the lines. In pain I recall writhing on the floor begging for someone, anyone, to come to my rescue and end my suffering. In darkness and confusion I have hoped for someone, anyone, to shine a tiny glimmer of light into my darkness, so that I might find a way. In anger and fury I have cursed every living thing, for not hearing my cries. (1989, p. 4)

Women of color in Los Angeles became the largest and most cohesive DSIN chapter in the United States. Their shared stories culminated in a realization that Harbor General Hospital and the Women's Clinic in Los Angeles were among the earliest sites where thousands of women were fitted with the Shield. Their experiences parallel the traumatic effects of the early birth control pill trials among Puerto Rican women, who were also abused by not being informed about the experimental nature of their participation (Mintz, 1967).

Among the compounded insults and obstacles that women of color faced are the lack of access to quality health care when their injuries manifested, the lack of publicity in their communities about their rights to file claims in Richmond, and their inability to acquire the medical documentation to support their claims for compensation now from the Dalkon Shield Claimants Trust.

Vera Davis, the Los Angeles coordinator of DSIN, noted the total absence of publicity in the African-American media about filing claims. During 1988 and 1989, she initiated an extraordinary effort in her local press to inform African-American women of their rights to file claims. She was overwhelmed by the thousands of women who responded to her telephone helpline. At this point, the best these women could hope for was a successful petition to make a "late claim," since the deadline for claims was in 1987.

Many Los Angeles women who joined DSIN in 1988 shared stories of doctors refusing to give them their records, even in cases where records still existed. Record keeping by their service providers was slipshod and inadequate, particularly in public assistance clinics. Davis also dramatized the problem of clinic and hospital closings and relocations, often due to fiscal distress, urban renewal, and redevelopment. She compiled a list of 29 hospitals in greater Los Angeles that were operating in the 1970s but have since closed. In 1989, a newspaper announced the closing of 13 women's and family-planning clinics in Los Angeles (Garcia, 1989). For the most part, however, the long gap of time assured that medical records would be lost, purged, or destroyed. By a strange coincidence, about a year earlier, in February 1989, one of the largest medical records storage buildings for Harbor General Hospital burned to the ground the evening following a large, publicized DSIN meeting at which national leaders were in attendence.

The Los Angeles chapter of DSIN began encouraging women to do their own research and teaching them how to go after copies of their records. These women organized a protest march at Harbor General Hospital in April 1990, to which the local media were invited. Hospital authorities were rattled at the bad press and made a public effort to give out records while the television cameras rolled on. Women in the Los Angeles chapter of DSIN also reported that insurance companies and public assistance agencies were requiring them to sign liens against their eventual settlements. Signing the liens was a condition of the women's getting their medical records, without which they cannot receive proper settlements from the Trust. The agencies are using the enforced liens in an attempt to recover monies they paid out for women's medical expenses related to their Shield injuries. Additionally, these women lack access to higher-quality legal assistance to help them negotiate the rigorous and tricky process of gaining compensation from the Trust.

Of the original 332,000 claims sent in to the Richmond Bankruptcy Court, some 135,000 women were excluded in 1987 for failing to comply with court-imposed deadlines for the submission of an official questionnaire. Data analysis of that large, excluded group would be compelling. I hypothesize that women of color and women from other countries were disproportionately excluded from the original group, relative to middle-class, white U.S. women. Anecdotal information collected in letters, telephone calls, and structured interviews suggests that many women of color, particularly those of low socioeconomic status, suffered significantly worse medical and legal treatment.

Among Katie Falls's writings during her DSIN activism is the following poem, which takes a partial look at the particular abuse of African-American women.

Where's My Purple Heart?
I was young, black, and female
    An American, most of all
I was proudly studying for success
    when I was drafted for The Cause.
I was an unwilling participant
    but I wore that IUD
I marched with my flags in hand
    because I was drafted to the Cause.
There was rights for blacks and women
    mainly for Population Control
My flag bore a crab-like thing
    I was drafted to the cause.
But as it tore away at me
    and I could no longer fight
They turned from me and laughed at me
    those who had drafted me to The Cause.
Now many years have past
    who I was, has long since gone
My flag is now Yellow, Red and Black
    but WHERE'S MY PURPLE HEART?

Women in Other Countries

The extent of the social control of contraception by population control agencies in third-world countries has been documented by Hartmann (1987). In the early 1980s, political authorities in Indonesia even held events called "IUD smiling safaris." At towns all over Java and Bali, local bigwigs (men) in safari suits greeted women, who were herded into tents for "indoctrination." Women who accepted the IUD were called *aspari* (angels) and given four kilos of rice after being inserted with an IUD. Observers likened this event to a religious crusade. USAID officials were invited to attend the event.

Hartmann describes the "machine model" of family planning in many third-world countries, where filling quotas, meeting targets, and supervisors enforcing the programs are commonplace. According to a chart published by Worldwatch, more than 12 third-world countries offer "incentives" to individuals who agree to either sterilization or contraceptives, and more than 17 third-world countries give incentives to either doctors or family-planning workers (Jacobsen, 1983).

Despite the special dangers inherent in high-tech contraception in low-tech environments, the use of IUDs is favored. Even Tietze, the population control scientist and a fervent advocate for the global adoption of IUDs, admits to the problems of lack of documentation on outcome abroad:

> I have no doubt but there must have been deaths associated with IUDs in Pakistan villages, and so forth. The medical systems of these countries are not so constructed that these things come to attention. (Committee on Government Operations, 1973, p. 375)

It is entirely likely that women in other countries, particularly third-world countries, suffered dramatically worse results with the Dalkon Shield than most U.S. women. The greatest potential for danger comes from at least four sources: (1) Shields shipped abroad were not packaged individually in a sterile environment; in fact, they were thrown into cardboard boxes, with only one inserter stick for every 1,000 devices; (2) the training for proper insertion and removal could only have been inferior, since the sparse copies of instruction pamphlets accompanying boxes were written only in English; (3) the clinics women visited when they experienced problems were ill equipped to treat or even recognize damages correctly; and (4) local family planning agencies that were committed to the use of IUDs would resist publicizing the issue at all, as discussed above. In all likelihood, death rates for these women were considerably higher than for U.S. women, as acknowledged even by population control experts. Morton Mintz addresses this issue: "Eighteen deaths have been reported, but the toll is certainly much higher, if only because in Third-World countries, no one was counting" (1991, p. 66).

Dalkon Shield activists have received reports that women were still being implanted with Shields well into the 1980s, with multiple reports from Latin America and Africa. Martina Langley, an attorney in Austin, Texas, has written repeatedly to the Richmond Bankruptcy Court officials, citing her first-hand observation of women getting Dalkon Shields in Central America in the 1980s during her time working in a family-planning clinic in Guatemala. Langley has been trying desperately to get court and population officials in USAID to respond to the unfair treatment of these women.

The Central American Experience. Langley has compiled and circulated handwritten letters from women who were coerced into using Shields, who were told it was a good product, and who were threatened and intimidated into keeping quiet and not pressing any claims of injury (after the notification program from the bankruptcy proceedings began). Translated excerpts of these letters written by Central American women include the following:

> Many women are afraid because when they go to APROFAN [clinic], they tell us we are lying, and then they said they do not have any records because they got burned or lost, and we feel helpless after listening to all this. (Guatemalan woman, personal communication, 1987)

> When I went to the clinic, they told me they were not able to give me any papers . . . and I could be lying . . . and the device never caused problems. . . . Look at this nurse . . . she wears one without any problems. (Salvadoran woman, personal communication, 1987)

> Although I remained under the ADS [Asociación Demográfica Salvadoreña] care all these years, they never told me that the Dalkon Shield should be removed, and for this reason I say they are very deficient. (Salvadoran woman, personal communication, 1987)

In Costa Rica, public health officials claim no women there had ill effects, even though Langley had personal contact with injured women and helped many of them to submit claims to the Richmond Bankruptcy Court around 1987. Local doctors, as reported in a newspaper article on this subject, proclaimed that Costa Rican women suffered no damages and were not at risk for injury from the Dalkon Shield because they "differ in physical profile and sexual conduct from their North American counterparts" (Shallat, 1987, p. 5a).

According to Langley, not one penny was spent in Central America to notify women of their right to file claims. (A. H. Robins spent nearly $5 million in the United States to notify women in the 1980s.) "When the company offered to make a similar publicity campaign in the Central American countries, the response was that there was no need, as the women had already removed it" (Langley, personal communication, 1988). When she personally hung up posters in Central American health clinics with warnings and a picture of the Shield, they were torn down. Langley claims USAID officials told her that their commitment in general to IUDs precludes them from supporting "any activity with a negative overall effect on their family planning effort" (Shallat, 1987, p. 5a). Her overall experience trying to get current information to women and health care workers in Central

America led her to a cynical conclusion, evidenced in her letter to the then-director of population for USAID:

> It is my belief that the ignorance of medical entities funded by your agency is not confined to the Dalkon Shield, but encompasses the total spectrum of contraceptives and is not limited to Central America geographically. (Personal communication, February 29, 1988)

The African Experience. Numerous reports of comparable experiences emanate from different parts of Africa. A former Dalkon Shield user and piano teacher writes from South Africa:

> I teach two daughters of a woman doctor who tells me she remembers inserting the Dalkon Shield into women as late as 1981!!!! When I questioned her about this, she said it was only for certain "selected patients" but how the selection was made I didn't ascertain. (P. Ackhurst, personal communication, June 7, 1987)

A female physician from Central Africa (Tanzania) wrote to DSIN, claiming that "information about the Dalkon Shield is scanty in my country, although it is still being used widely" (Dr. A. Kiwara, personal communication, June 16, 1987). A family-planning specialist wrote from Dakar that she had worked in that clinic since 1976 and had her own Dalkon Shield removed in 1980 (M. B. Baye, personal communication, October 14, 1987). Attorney Shainwald attended the major global conference on women held in Nairobi in 1986 and held a press conference about the Dalkon Shield there. Women who attended knew next to nothing about the damages associated with the Shield and virtually nothing about the court proceedings against the company.

Pleas for a Worldwide Recall. A few years earlier, in 1983, Robert Manchester, a Vermont attorney, had submitted a citizen's petition to the FDA for a worldwide recall. This effort resulted in Manchester's direct negotiations with the Robins Company to implement most of the items he asked for in that petition. Letters were sent to embassies abroad, leaving notification of those women to the local authorities. Substantially more money was spent to notify U.S. women. The countries with the largest response to this recall were the countries where women's rights and women's health organizations played an active role, taking the initiative to notify women in their countries. For example, in Canada, the Vancouver Women's Health Collective made a valiant attempt to publicize this case. In Australia, the women's group Fertility Action undertook to publicize the recall. In the United Kingdom, the Women's Reproductive Health and Information Centre has been active. In Ireland, the Council on the Status of Women played a role. In the Netherlands, consumer health organizations are credited with notifying Dalkon Shield users.

DSIN's attempts to enlist the help of WHO in organizing a worldwide recall campaign around 1988 failed. For this initiative, DSIN was able to gain the support and co-advocacy of some international consumer-based health organizations. Most notable were the efforts of Health Action International (HAI) and the Women's Global Network for Reproductive Rights (based in the Netherlands) in circulating petitions to their sister regional organizations around the world. These groups returned signed petitions from women in about 30 different countries. Also, HAI representatives assisted DSIN in framing our request to WHO. Both agencies also sent supporting letters directly to WHO, imploring a recall.

Dr. M. F. Fathalla, WHO's director of a special program of research in human reproduction, responded in typical bureaucratic fashion to the DSIN request:

> If, as you say, some women were still using the "Dalkon Shield," they would be outside the reach of the normal information channels. Under its Constitution, WHO is not permitted to take direct action in its Member States unless they ask it to do so. (personal communication, November 15, 1989)

Few Claims from Non-U.S. Women. When the notification campaign to locate potential Dalkon Shield claimants was ordered by the bankruptcy court in 1985, only a fraction of money was spent abroad, as already noted. As a result, only a fraction of all claims are from non-U.S. women. Attorney Manchester filed a petition with the Richmond Bankruptcy Court in 1985, requesting that *equal* notice be given or sent to women abroad.

In 1987, DSIN leaders discussed the lack of notification to women abroad during a visit to Mike Sheppard, then the Clerk of the bankruptcy court. Sheppard produced a computer printout of all claims submitted to the court as of February 1987. This computer record shows a total of 332,673 claims received by that date, with 180,055 completed questionnaires returned to the court. There were 32,222 international claims from 101 countries; however, only 18,689 questionnaires were returned to the court. This is an approximate ratio of 10 U.S. claims to 1 foreign claim, despite the estimate that around 1.7 million women abroad—a number nearly equal to that of U.S. women—also used the device. Manchester's earlier petition to the FDA for a recall included sales figures for the device abroad (see Table 2.1).

The distribution of the device abroad and the number of claims submitted deserve comment. The largest number of international claims come from North American and European countries (see Table 2.2). The United Kingdom has 3,494 claims, the Netherlands 1,473, Australia 5,049, and Canada 3,027. Most of the third-world countries list claims in single or double digits only. There are several ways to account for this discrepancy. One is the fact that most of the women in these North American and European countries are represented legally by some of the top Dalkon Shield attorneys, who have traveled to the Western countries mentioned above. Second, the organized women's rights and consumer health groups in the North American and European countries were able to publicize the legal action so that thousands of women in those countries were sufficiently informed to submit claims of injury. Finally, women in third-world countries claim that their governments repressed the information or even

TABLE 2.1 Distribution of the Dalkon Shield Abroad

1970-1974 (from Robins sales records)	
South America	205,520
Southwest Asia and Africa	177,736
Europe	508,016
East Asia	153,480
TOTAL	1,044,752
1970-1974 Distributed through USAID (from General Services Administration)[a]	708,568
Known total of Dalkon Shields distributed abroad	**1,753,320**

Note: Data obtained from Robert Manchester, Esq., *Citizen's Petition to the FDA*, April 1983.
[a]Geographical breakdown not available.

TABLE 2.2 Number of Official Claims, by Region, as of 5 Feb. 1987

The Americas (not U.S./Canada)		Southwest Asia and Africa		Europe		East Asia	
Argentina	43	Botswana	3	Austria	8	Australia	5049
Bahamas	11	Cameroon	1	Belgium	39	Bangladesh	52
Belize	2	Egypt	3	Denmark	85	India	55
Brazil	1135	Ethiopia	3	W. Germany	260	Japan	8
Chile	2	Iran	4	Finland	79	Malaysia	9
Colombia	18	Israel	236	France	105	New Zealand	474
Costa Rica	56	Kenya	32	Greece	17	Pakistan	6
Dominican Rep.	5	Kuwait	1	Iceland	1	Papua N. Guinea	8
Ecuador	6	Lesotho	4	Ireland	349	Philippines	508
El Salvador	31	Liberia	2	Italy	27	Singapore	1
Grenada	1	Malawi	2	Luxemborg	2	Sri Lanka	14
Guatemala	15	Nigeria	30	Malta	2	Taiwan	696
Honduras	2	Oman	1	Netherlands	1473	Thailand	3
Jamaica	15	Saudi Arabia	10	Norway	254	Vanuatu	1
Mexico	15	S. Africa	283	Poland	2	Vietnam	1
Nicaragua	6	Swaziland	2	Portugal	3	W. Samoa	1
Panama	13	Syria	2	Spain	11	TOTAL	6886
Paraguay	2	Tanzania	3	Sweden	479		
Peru	1	Tonga	2	Switzerland	6		
Trinidad	2	Tunisia	2	U.K.	3494		
Venezuela	1	Turkey	28	Yugoslavia	1		
TOTAL	1382	Uganda	2	TOTAL	6697		
		U.A.E.	4				
		Zaire	1				
		Zambia	6				
		Zimbabwe	19				
		TOTAL	686				

All original claims from the following countries did not comply with Bankruptcy Court protocol and were thereby summarily denied: Algeria, Antigua, Barbados, Central African Republic, Gambia, Ghana, Haiti, Indonesia, South Korea, St. Vincent, Sudan

Total number of international claims as of 5 Feb. 1987 (including Canada, with 3027 claims): 18,689

Total number of U.S. claims as of 2 Feb. 1987: 161,351

Source: Data obtained from U.S. Bankruptcy Court, Richmond, VA.

actively intimidated women into not pressing forward. These governments were anxious not to disrupt their political ties to the United
States and its agencies, such as USAID.

Constance Miller, a Dalkon Shield activist in Seattle, has spoken
with South Korean women and their attorneys, many of whose claims
were discounted early on by the court. The sole reason for denying
their claims was procedural, according to Miller: The court misspelled
many names, which delayed the timely receipt of the official questionnaire. Additionally, documents from the court were mailed at
surface rate—not air mail—which caused them to miss the court-
imposed deadline. Attorneys who requested the inclusion of these
types of cases were told by the court that it could not make excep-
tions for individuals. Sybil Shainwald, a New York attorney, reports
similar frustrations in trying to help women from India. With incomplete addresses and the court-imposed deadline, it became impossible
to register many Indian claims.

Articles published outside the United States and letters written
to DSIN point to the great frustration at this exclusion. Even women
as geographically close as Canada felt a chasm of isolation and moun-
tains of obstacles in getting claims information and in communicating with the bankruptcy court in Richmond. Women in Quebec who
were strongly allied with DSIN expressed great despair at the prospect
that they would have to pay huge sums just to have their records
translated into English. Attorney Manchester cites sales of 133,408
Dalkon Shields in Canada, yet only a trivial number of women were
ever informed enough to be able to file a claim. Nora Morin, one of
the Quebec activists, wrote early to DSIN, "I think Robins has succeeded
in intimidating most Canadian women (but not all of us). The bor-
der jitters I call it" (personal communication, September 14, 1987).

Another issue that compounded the difficulty in women's making claims occurred in the case of countries, religions, or ethnic groups
that banned or severely restricted contraception, for example, Ireland.
Some Irish women went to Great Britain to get their IUDs secretly.
According to attorney Manchester, who represents thousands of
women in Great Britain, Ireland, and Canada, the Shield was even
smuggled into Irish clinics for insertion. Obviously, keeping records
was impossible where contraception was illegal. When injuries manifested, women faced both medical and personal dilemmas about dis-
closing their actions. How could they tell doctors and how could they
expect to be included in the compensation scheme if it meant reveal-
ing this secret? (This issue has also surfaced in letters received from
Catholic women, especially from Hispanic cultures. Many of them did

not tell anyone, including their husbands, that they were using the device. Furthermore, many of these women were intensely anguished when they later discovered that this device is an abortifacient; that is, it can precipitate an abortion.)

Manchester reports extreme difficulty in locating medical records in Ireland because the health care system is poor in general and record keeping is almost nonexistent, particularly for women who could not afford private doctors. Manchester also found the Irish authorities extremely resistant to releasing records, even more so than in the United States. A U.S. newspaper article reports the inadequacy of the Irish Department of Health in informing persons of their rights to compensation ("Irishwomen to share," 1989). Langley and Shainwald also mentioned these problems in connection with countries in Latin America, South and Southwest Asia, and Africa.

Governments Resist Women's Claims. DSIN received a long letter from the Women's Health Information Center in Israel, describing the Israeli experience, which parallels those already cited. That women's organization decided to notify women on its own, due to the failure of the authorities to act.

> We knew that A. H. Robins Co. claimed to have sold the Dalkon Shield in Israel, but [Israeli medical authorities] had no idea of how many were actually inserted in Israeli women. The Ministry of Health told a reporter from a local newspaper that there were none in Israel. However, in mid-February we placed a small ad in the same newspaper and over 100 women responded immediately! (Women's Health Information Center, personal communication, October 1987)

The letter goes on to describe how women from every part of Israel eventually contacted the group and how the hospitals resisted cooperating to the point that many women were not able to file a claim in time. Records were spotty, incomplete, and missing. The women's group estimates that, at best, only half the number of users eligible for compensation actually were able to file a claim, due to resistance by the medical system.

The Bangladesh situation was extreme. Farhad Mazhar and Farida Akhter were staff members of UBINIG, a consumer organization there. Mazhar worked in the Policy Research for Development Alternatives branch. Around 1987, when they tried to advertise and notify Dalkon Shield users about their right to compensation, these consumer advocates were harassed by the government: Their offices were raided and they were arrested. The authorities saw this notification program as an anti-U.S. (and, therefore, pro-communist) threat. The government did not want to deal with the implications of how this health disaster had been allowed to happen. This situation came to light when Mazhar traveled to the United States and Canada to try to file claims and to meet with advocates for Dalkon Shield users in North America.

REVISING HISTORY

By 1991 medical journals were again publishing articles on the Dalkon Shield, suggesting that it really was a good contraceptive device. These new critics reproached the medical studies conducted in the 1970s, which had reported high rates of disease associated with the Shield relative to other IUDs. Kronmal, Whitney, and Mumford (1991) attacked the case-control methodology used in the Women's Health Study (Burkman, 1981; Lee, Rubin, Ory, & Burkman, 1983). In the abstract of his 1991 article, Kronmal acknowledges that he served as an expert witness for A. H. Robins during Shield-related court trials and that his newly published remarks were part of the work he did for them almost 10 years ago, when Robins was preparing its defense strategy in courts around the country. Kronmal's article hit the front page of the *New York Times* (Altman, 1991) and received wide attention in the popular press. That the Kronmal piece was widely misconstrued as *new* data was reflected in the titles of other news articles. A follow-up article titled "Dalkon Shield Trust Might Use New Data to Limit Some Payments" in the *Wall Street Journal* (Waldholz, 1991) reveals the underlying motivation for publishing these disputable findings. At this time, women who rejected the initial offers from the Trust were beginning to move ahead with jury trials around the United States.

> The release of Mr. Kronmal's sharply worded attack comes at an especially crucial time in the distribution of the [Dalkon Shield] trust fund. . . . Michael Sheppard, executive director of the trust, said the trust's legal counsel would use the new study's findings "on a case-by-case basis" if it helped to defend cases that went to arbitration or to court. Mr. Kronmal said he has been asked by the trust to testify in future hearings, adding that he has agreed to testify if asked. (Waldholz, 1991, p. B2)

This circumstance pushes the threshold of speculation and conjecture about just how much the medical profession colludes with corporate medical interests to preserve its own interests. That medical journals publish such questionable work, in this calculated fashion, should give rise to an investigation into the connections and relationships among medical researchers such as Kronmal, pharmaceutical companies, and medical journal editors. This issue should also be included in the discourse of medical ethicists who are currently examining the medical research enterprise in response to increasing charges of falsification of experimental data.

Mumford and Kessel (1992) then published an article, also assailing the Women's Health Study methodology. Their motivation for doing so, in my opinion, indicates a conjuncture of interests with advocates of population control:

> Because of the indictment of the Dalkon Shield, both clinicians and the public have developed strongly negative perceptions of IUDs in general that are not improving with the passage of time. Rehabilitation of the IUD contraceptive method in the United States cannot be effected if these Dalkon Shield–related negative perceptions persist. (p. 1151)

Furthermore, their views appear to ignore or even to deny history:

> The 71 clinical trials of the Dalkon Shield show that when this device is inserted by an experienced clinician it is a safe and effective contraceptive method, comparable with other IUDs used at the time. . . . This study offers convincing evidence that the indictment of the Dalkon Shield was a mistake. (p. 1151)

Dr. David Eschenbach (1920), a respected gynecologist who researches and publishes widely on pelvic inflammatory disease and IUDs, takes issue with his colleagues and these "new" studies in his role as editor for the journal *Fertility and Sterility*:

> The timing of the reviews 17 years after the Dalkon Shield was removed from the market may be perplexing to some, but not to the women who are now filing court claims. . . . The two reviews presented such a one-sided view that they are best termed extensive editorials. (p. 1178)

SUMMARY

The material in this chapter adheres to the conflict-of-interest perspective on contraceptive technology and the impact of IUDs on women's health. High-status officials, such as pharmaceutical executives, physicians, and population scientists, have vast resources to propagate their version of the "truth" or the "facts." Evidence amassed against great odds by the victims themselves contradicts the "benevolence" of prevailing economic and social arrangements (Kidder & Fine, 1986, p. 56). In this case, the commitment of population control agencies to disseminate high-tech contraception has had unconscionable costs— all to the women who are individually "expendable in the general scheme of things," from the experts' perspective. It is by unearthing these contradictions that social problems can be redefined in order to provoke social change.

3 Chronology of the Dalkon Shield Information Network

This chapter documents the embryonic stages of the Dalkon Shield Information Network from 1987 to 1989 and focuses on the critical events and issues that shaped the group's development. Appendix B summarizes the chronological developments both at court and within DSIN. Representative comments from other Dalkon Shield women are cited from among the more than 400 unsolicited letters sent by Dalkon Shield survivors to DSIN or by women's names, if they are DSIN chapter leaders. Ten chapter leaders were interviewed for this research about their roles in DSIN.

This chapter occasionally refers to three other Dalkon Shield advocacy groups, but the history and internal relations of those groups are not the subjects of this research. The relations among all the Dalkon Shield advocacy groups is discussed in Chapter 4.

THE CULTURE OF SILENCE

Except for a handful of anecdotal stories in the popular press during the 1970s and 1980s, Dalkon Shield users did not speak out or attempt to organize until 1986, some 18 years after the early injuries. Although approximately 9,500 women received financial settlements totaling $530 million by August 1985, only a few women had ever spoken out publicly about their experiences up to this date. At the time Robins filed for Chapter 11 protection in 1985, about 6,000 lawsuits were pending, with an average of 15 lawsuits being filed every day.

During the first one and a half years of bankruptcy proceedings before DSIN was founded, the only information available to women about the progress of the case was an occasional story discreetly tucked into the business pages of several large newspapers, such as the *Wall Street Journal*, the *New York Times*, or the *Washington Post*. Then, in 1986, the Robins Company was forced to comply with a court-ordered media publicity campaign to advise Dalkon Shield users that they could file claims against Robins. By the time DSIN organized formally in January 1987, more than 332,000 injury claims had been filed at the Richmond court. However, the only contact these women had from the court was a postcard acknowledging receipt of their claim, assigning them a claim number, and bearing the admonition, "Do not contact this court for information."[1]

Awareness of Injustice

My own need for information became pressing to me after I was asked to appear on a Philadelphia talk show with author Susan Perry in October 1985 to promote her new book, *Nightmare: Women and the Dalkon Shield*. Sybil Shainwald, a women's health activist, lawyer, and former president of the board of directors of the National Women's Health Network (NWHN), had contacted me about appearing on this show. I had become acquainted with Shainwald from reading the NWHN newsletter (see the section below entitled "Seeking Support and Assistance").

Although I already had hired a lawyer to represent my own personal-injury case (before the Robins bankruptcy petition froze all litigation), this television experience in 1985 was the context in which I discovered the origin and cause of the tragedy. I was enraged that Dr. Hugh Davis (the inventor of this device), the Robins Company, and the Aetna Insurance Company had concealed from me and almost 4 million other women vital information that could have prevented the mass injuries. In fact, this discovery made me emotionally ill with a deep depression for several weeks. Many other women comment that acquiring this information represented a dramatic, pivotal point for them, too. Letter #284 states: "After reading the articles you sent me, I now know that I am one among many women who have been victimized by a predominately male, greed-ruled company that our culture still upholds." Another woman expressed similar feelings in an interview:

> I had no yen to sue for vengeance—until a 1985 *Washington Post* series by Morton Mintz told me how much the Robins company already knew about the dangers of the shield when it was peddled to me as "the ideal new contraceptive." (Breslin, 1989, p. 49)

By the time this information finally became available to them, many women had already spent years suffering with various illnesses

and, obviously, without correct, adequate diagnoses for their maladies.

> For years, the doctor continually told me that I was the only one
> who ever complained. He wondered what my problem was. It was
> so belittling that I thought it must be me. (Sherry Fletcher)

> It should be noted that I am not looking for money, but an answer
> to the question "Why Me?" It was a long mental recovery but
> never knowing why was the worst of it. (Letter #300)

For all these years, many women perceived their problems as
idiosyncratic misfortunes. Many blamed themselves for their injuries.
Kidder and Fine (1986) have noted previously how many instances
of social injustice are kept private. (The sociopolitical implications of
this silence were addressed in Chapter 2.) In the Dalkon Shield case,
the sexual implications of contraception presented an additional significant barrier that women had to break through in order publicly
to advocate their own rights. This was even more difficult for women
who had used the Shield without telling their partners, husbands,
families, gynecologists, or family doctors. There were many women
whose religious convictions prohibited birth control methods with
abortifacient properties, such as the IUD, and who thus felt compelled
to keep their use of contraception a private matter.

Many of the women who contacted DSIN were engulfed in a victim-blaming ideology. In the earliest lawsuits against Robins, the
company's defense lawyers attacked women's sexual histories and
tried to build a case that their injuries were the result of venereal disease caused by their "promiscuity" and poor "hygiene." The link
between injury and sexuality exacerbated the feelings of personal fault,
even though Robins's explanation has been rejected everywhere else.
In many of the early lawsuits, Robins's defense lawyers cross-exam-
ined women during trials, eliciting explicit details of their sexual
behavior, such as who their partners were and whether they engaged
in oral and anal sex. This deeply humiliating exposure prevented many
women from pressing forward with personal-injury lawsuits.

Sadly, many injured women did not receive validation from any
quarter. In fact, other people in their social web (including family
members, mental health workers, and doctors) functioned as pawns
in promoting victim-blaming ideologies and convinced them that they
were angry, crazy, fragile, or overly sensitive (Kidder & Fine, 1986).

I felt upon reading the articles you sent me that I am not alone in my anger, the frustration, or that I was damned by God to be infertile. (Letter #284)

The financial award is insult [added] to injury. Loss of faith in the medical world, loss of faith in your own body, loss of faith in your self-worth. (Letter #333)

I am grateful that at least I know what is wrong with me now. When I didn't know, I really felt like I was crazy. (Letter #210)

After reading the Morton Mintz and Susan Perry books, I felt both raging anger and yet relief. The anger—that a corporation could do these things and get away with it. The relief—knowing that I wasn't crazy. (Letter #413)

Conscientizacao

Self-awareness is critical to the process of transforming self from passive object into active subject (Freire, 1970). People will take action against the oppressive elements of their reality only when they struggle and learn to perceive social, political, and economic contradictions. This is the process that Paolo Freire calls *conscientizacao*. Even if some individual Dalkon Shield women perceived the grave injustice done to them, they were still virtually isolated from others and needed a mechanism for linking their circumstances to those of other victims. Gloria Manago commented, "Before I found your group, I had been fighting this man [Davis] all the time, but alone, within my heart."

Once awareness of the true cause for the injuries was heightened, some Dalkon Shield women began to feel anger, then rage. Early DSIN members expressed anger about several specific issues: (1) the betrayal of trust by the medical system that caused their senseless, needless suffering; (2) the loss of their reproductive potential and the violation of their bodily integrity; and (3) their perception that officials of A. H. Robins escaped full accountability by hiding in the bankruptcy system and by not being criminally prosecuted.

After reading Mintz's book recently, I started feeling a lot of anger, frustration, and sense of betrayed trust toward Robins. (Letter #202)

It really makes me mad when I think what Robins has done to thousands of women. It's the cause of nearly destroying my life.

After 13 years, I'm still suffering. I am unable to work. (Letter #214)

Seeking Support and Assistance

By mid-1986, I was keeping a crude index card file of names and facts that I gleaned from the newspaper articles relevant to the Dalkon Shield issue. I subscribed to the *Wall Street Journal*. I visited attorney Shainwald in order to read some of the Shield-related legal briefs and court documents.[2] It was only by examining these documents and questioning Shainwald that I discovered the existence of a court-appointed Dalkon Shield Claimants' Committee, our official representatives in the Richmond Bankruptcy Court, who formally negotiated on behalf of all Dalkon Shield claimants in the bankruptcy proceedings.

The prospect of locating and informing thousands of other women was a staggering undertaking, so I appealed to established organizations for help. I first wrote to Resolve, Inc., a national infertility organization, and to the National Women's Health Network, the organization Shainwald urged me to approach for advice and support. Women at Resolve headquarters were very encouraging and mentioned us in their newsletters to aid in our search for other Dalkan Shield users. Resolve had heard from many women injured by the Shield who were suffering infertility problems at that time. Women who read the Resolve newsletters began calling DSIN. At about the same time, Sherry Fletcher, another emerging DSIN leader, began contacting public interest health organizations in Michigan, where she lived.

I wrote to NWHN, suggesting the formation of a subcommittee to monitor Dalkon Shield developments and volunteering to work on this project with them. I reasoned that the long involvement of NWHN on behalf of Dalkon Shield users, coupled with their wealth of experience in championing women's health rights, made the group a natural ally. I also believed that such an alliance would be mutually beneficial, with the possibility of a large infusion of new members to NWHN from the large, presently unserved population of Dalkon Shield users.

Shainwald's encouragement aside, I never received a response to three letters I sent to Victoria Leonard, NWHN's executive director, over the course of many months. Eventually, Fletcher and I wrote a letter to their board of directors and were encouraged by Shainwald to attend a board meeting to seek NWHN's support and endorsement for our first Richmond rally in July 1987. They also promised to mention DSIN in their newsletter in the future. No agreement was ever reached about taking on this cause under their auspices in the manner we had hoped. Fletcher and I reached the conclusion that we would have to champion the Dalkon Shield cause independently of NWHN. We could waste no more time. (See the section entitled "The Women's Health Movement Organizations" in Chapter 4 for a description of the dynamic of social relations.)

After this outreach attempt failed, I wrote a proposal outline to the Dalkon Shield Claimants' Committee, appointed by the bankruptcy court to represent all claimants in Richmond, suggesting the formation of an information service for all Dalkon Shield claimants. The Claimants' Committee had five members, three of whom were women claimants. Two of those women were bankruptcy lawyers. The Committee was represented by the Washington, DC, law firm of Cadwalader, Wickersham, and Taft. I never received a response to my proposal from anyone, and, in fact, I have no idea what happened to that document. Months later, after I established communication with one of the claimant members of the Committee, that woman told me she had never received the proposal.

In June 1986, I had sent the same proposal to Robert R. Merhige, Jr., the judge presiding over the bankruptcy proceedings, again suggesting that a support and information network be established by the court to aid the victims during the lengthy legal proceeding that had frozen all personal-injury litigation. I never received a reply, and I do not know why.

Fletcher and I became discouraged about getting moral or financial support for this project. At this time, I was too unfamiliar with these kinds of activities to know that follow-up telephone calls and some degree of badgering or hustling might help or hasten decision making. We were unaware at this time that another group was in the process of forming.

Information and the DSIN Newsletter

Fletcher and I continued to consult with Shainwald. She encouraged us to form our own group, using the phrase "Don't agonize; organize!" I began publishing a newsletter from my home in Bethlehem, Pennsylvania, in January 1987, with a meager list of names and addresses from Shainwald's personal contacts with other Dalkon Shield users. About 20 women sent a $5 subscription fee, launching DSIN. After a newspaper article appeared in the Allentown, Pennsylvania, newspaper, several local women contacted me and began to volunteer, compiling a mailing list and mailing the newsletters.

The early goal of DSIN was to become a source of emotional support to women. Part of that included providing credible, correct, and detailed information about the case and its impact on the women whose lives were wrapped up in it. To do this effectively, DSIN needed to establish legitimacy as quickly as possible. Early advice from experienced grass-roots organizers was that incorporating as a nonprofit organization would give DSIN the formal identity it needed for credibility. So, by a simple bureaucratic procedure of filing an application with the state, we incorporated DSIN as a nonprofit organization at the outset.

The DSIN newsletter helped break the culture of silence in which these victims had lived for so many years:

> I am thrilled that I now can get information. Just to know that there are others out there with me and as outraged as I am about what was done to me [is a relief]. (Letter #242)

> I received your newsletter and was suddenly confronted with the reality that I am not alone. This is a strange and difficult realization, but it is also very healthy. (Letter #233)

As we discovered later, other women around the country were also trying to track the court developments through the national newspapers. As noted earlier, news about this case was restricted to the business pages, surfacing only with new developments in the bankruptcy negotiations. Women who eventually contacted DSIN by tracking down sporadic mention of the group in media stories reported that they were following the case in virtual isolation, completely on their own. Shirley Nichols commented, "I was interested in contacting *anybody* who could give me any information because I felt totally alone. I wanted to know what was happening. I wanted to know history; it was therapy for me."

With new information about the origins of the problems, women began to redefine what had happened as a public violation of basic human rights, not as a personal misfortune. The educational process triggered by DSIN activism began some women's transition from individual despair to a growing mass consciousness and awareness.

> Most frustrating is that there has been no opportunity for me to stand face to face with Mr. Robins and say "You took away my right to have a child." (Letter #329)

> Tell me, was Dr. Davis raped of his medical license just like so many women were raped of their rights as a mother and a woman? (Letter #333)

CONFRONTING THE SYSTEM

In my research for the newsletter, I traveled to Richmond to see Judge Merhige and several other people who were quoted regularly in newspaper accounts. I was especially interested in speaking with Dave Schiller, the U.S. Attorney for the state of Virginia, who was often quoted in the Richmond newspaper reports of the bankruptcy proceeding. He had boldly criticized Robins for delaying justice to the women.

Although I now felt rage toward Robins's executives from what I had learned, I was terrified about going to Richmond, Robins's corporate headquarters and hometown. Many DSIN leaders who also eventually traveled to Richmond felt the same fear, which we now jokingly refer to as the "Silkwood syndrome."[3] Richmond loomed ominously. I asked Cinders Murdock-Vaughan, a childhood friend recently rediscovered, to accompany me on that first trip. At that point, she knew virtually nothing about DSIN or my activities. As a result of our conversations on the trip, she discovered that her own unhappy history of reproductive damage, which included PID, infertility, and a hysterectomy at the age of 27, could have been due to the fact that she also had used the Dalkon Shield. Murdock-Vaughan went with me on almost every subsequent trip and became the vice-president of DSIN.

Naively, I had not scheduled appointments with anyone for this first trip. When we entered Judge Merhige's chambers, his law clerk told us that the judge could not meet with *litigants*. I had no idea what a *litigant* was! We were able to meet with an associate of U.S. Attorney Schiller, who explained what specific issues of justice their staff was working on. We also met with Mike Sheppard, then clerk of the U.S. Bankruptcy Court, who was in charge of storing and handling all the Dalkon Shield records. Judge Merhige would later appoint Sheppard the executive director of the Dalkon Shield Claimants Trust.

We were eager to know how to enlarge our mailing list with names and addresses of other claimants from the court records. Sheppard told us that the records were under court seal and thus not available to the public. We were still so unfamiliar with the entire court process that we only discovered days later that women from another newly formed Dalkon Shield organization and their lawyers were also in town that day for a court hearing, precisely to argue the question of public access to the claimant mailing list! We also had no idea at this time that this other group had the great fortune to be assisted by Alan Morrison, attorney and the head of litigation for Public Citizen, one of Ralph Nader's consumers' rights organizations. At that time, we did not appreciate the importance of that connection. It is difficult to get *pro bono* assistance from lawyers in a case as complex as this one.

REFRAMING ROBINS'S STORY

The more I learned about what is involved in bankruptcy proceedings, the more insatiable my appetite for information became. To me, the proceedings appeared stalled: more than a year had passed, but nothing significant was happening in Richmond.[4] The court had already granted to A. H. Robins many extensions on its submission of a reorganization plan, which is the resolution of a Chapter 11 proceeding. Early in 1987, American Home Products (AHP) made its first bid to buy A. H. Robins in a cash deal, but that negotiation failed, primarily because Robins's executives wanted the lucrative severance packages often called "golden parachutes." I was angered by that story in the *Wall Street Journal* (Waldholz & Freedman, 1987). When the judge granted yet another delay later that year, I became even angrier.

I also learned that the Robins Company was not bankrupt. I discovered this news by reading the *Wall Street Journal* accounts and the Robins annual shareholder reports as part of my own background research. This news was a revelation. Robins was, in fact, a financially robust, multinational pharmaceutical company, with profits growing in every fiscal quarter, cash on hand, and little corporate debt. The subsidiaries of Robins were not part of the Chapter 11 filing, according to the *Wall Street Journal*. Robins's net profits were actually *rising* while under Chapter 11 status. E. C. Robins, Jr., president of the company, defended the Chapter 11 filing in a *Wall Street Journal* interview as necessary "to protect the company's vitality against those who would destroy it for the benefit of a few" (Schwadel, 1985, p. A3). I concluded that Robins was in the bankruptcy court not because it was bankrupt, but because it sought a mechanism to protect and preserve its substantial corporate assets.

Although there was an official legal process, I began to understand that the system was working to protect Robins's corporate interests to the detriment of the injured parties.[5] In sum, Chapter 11 was a business deal, from my perspective, and was not at all about justice. Other DSIN leaders remarked:

> Bankruptcy was just a maneuver to save as much as they could. They're hiding between the pages of our legal system. (Donna Reeck)

I thought it was just a big kangaroo court, just put us through the motions to make it look like justice was done. (Joanne Ackerman)

In 1988, a new DSIN leader in Colorado attended an information session for lawyers so that she could learn more about the case. She shared her observations about that meeting in her interview for this research:

It seemed so sterile in a way. They were talking about these little rules. . . . It just seemed so impersonal and so far removed from what it was really all about . . . the injustice and the corporate responsibility. (Jan Thompson)

Impetus for Action

Reframing the litigation in this context mobilized me and others into taking action. The DSIN newsletter began to report events from this perspective. Now I began calling women who subscribed to the newsletter, explaining the events in this way and asking them if they felt that a protest action on the courthouse steps was in order. There was much enthusiasm for such an event. Many more women began to volunteer their time and energy toward making a protest action a reality.

In sum, we emerged as a social movement when we defined our condition as an intolerable injustice rather than as a misfortune warranting charitable consideration (Ruzek, 1978). A perception of injustice as a collective problem enables people to fight for outcomes they themselves will control rather than to ask for help, which is controlled by authorities (Kidder & Fine 1986).

Naming the Injustice

Murdock-Vaughan and I made four trips to Richmond to prepare for the July 1987 Richmond rally, which was the first public gathering of Dalkon Shield survivors. On one of those early planning trips, we insisted on meeting with the legal counsel to the official Dalkon Shield Claimants' Committee, at the firm's offices in Washington, D.C. An associate at that law firm met with us briefly but would not divulge any information about the status of the sensitive negotiations at that time. He commented to the effect that his firm hoped things would be wrapped up soon, because it was not making the profit margin that it had anticipated for handling this case. In addition to the media-reported comments from Robins's officials about the business concerns, this comment from our chief advocate in the courtroom distressed us. It contributed to our understanding that this was a business deal and that the human dimensions of the case were of subordinate importance. The meeting left us with an urgent need to become more directly involved.

During this time, the claimants' mailing list became available to the public, due to the court motion of Alan Morrison on behalf of the other group. The stipulations, however, were daunting. Interested parties could either go to the court and hand-copy names and addresses from the individual file folders or pay 65 cents *per name* for a computer search and printout. The price was outrageously high, and most of the money would reimburse the Robins Company directly for contributing computer support to the court! Apparently, the court was not financially equipped to handle the staggering number of claims. DSIN did not have funds to purchase the list, so we determined to copy the names by hand. Ultimately, five people took turns at the records center, laboriously copying approximately 1,200 names and addresses directly onto mailing labels.[6]

The Victims Speak Out for the First Time

On July 21, 1987, a group of about 70 men and women demonstrated in front of the Richmond courthouse during a Shield-related court hearing, then marched en masse to the YWCA for a rally. In advance of the rally, women in contact with DSIN were electrified by the prospect of finally making a public challenge to the Robins Company. When the day of the rally came, however, some speakers and participants were apprehensive about mounting a public protest. We were totally inexperienced "organizers." It was the collective bond that gave the group courage to picket in front of the courthouse and to face the television cameras.

Many people from local Richmond groups participated in this protest action. In particular, women of color who were longtime local activists in the human rights community turned out to support this effort. These women, most of whom belonged to the Black Women's Political Network, had been the most helpful to us during the planning stages, and many showed up for the protest march. Their support and encouragement bolstered our courage. Other supporters included Diana Scully, a leading women's health care critic and professor at Virginia Commonwealth University in Richmond; Julie Lapham, then director of Richmond's Common Cause office; Lynn

Bradford, the head of the Richmond National Organization for Women (NOW); and Wendy Northrup, organizer of a local peace and justice group.

The local press coverage was substantial, both in the newspapers and on all the television channels. Dalkon Shield developments had made daily news in the Richmond press for several years, but this was the first time the Richmond community got a look at self-identified Dalkon Shield women.[7] Only two Dalkon Shield users from Richmond came out publicly. Many of them supported in spirit what we were doing but felt too vulnerable to go public.

In addition to publicizing the survivors' stories, DSIN announced a proactive agenda for the future, including campaigns for a formal product recall of the Shield, a criminal investigation of Robins's officers, a congressional investigation of the FDA for its failures in this matter, and the establishment of regional DSIN chapters. The rally slogan, "No more Shields for Robins' profits" remained highly visible throughout the bankruptcy proceedings. The written materials for the rally established DSIN's shift from information to direct political action.

> Dalkon Shield survivors will not tolerate any longer the stalling tactics that delay a just resolution to this catastrophe. Dalkon Shield survivors will meet to formulate their own strategy for bringing an end to the continuing pain and suffering inflicted by the bankruptcy proceeding.

Our use of the term *survivor* was also a conscious attempt to create the sense of activism and power necessary to effect change. DSIN leaders using the term *survivor* met with philosophical challenge from other groups and DSIN allies, who insisted that the term *victim* would garner more sympathy and support for the cause. Many DSIN members, however, expressed gratitude at the use of the term *survivor* as a more positive term that imparted a sense of personal power.

Media Appeals

After the first seven months, this embryonic organization could claim tangible achievements, including (1) three issues of the DSIN newsletter, (2) a successful protest action in Richmond, and (3) an action agenda with justice-oriented goals. There were now printed materials and newspaper stories to distribute to other organizations, Dalkon Shield women, and the national press.

The major obstacle at this time was DSIN's inability to reach large numbers of other women directly, so we made a deliberate attempt to draw national media attention. No one in DSIN had prior experience in public relations or media relations, but we learned quickly that becoming newsworthy demanded massive amounts of time and energy. We also discovered that taking action was the best way to get coverage, as opposed to just making announcements or comments. It was vital to craft focused, highly charged, and sharply critical messages, without being discounted or becoming objects of ridicule. Our first attempts were largely successful: DSIN spokespersons were quoted correctly, and many became credible personalities either in the national press or in their local regions. The press continually contacted them for comment on developments in the bankruptcy case. A press kit of informational materials was developed and sent out in response to all press inquiries, so that a reporter would have background material and the names of our contact persons at his or her fingertips when writing any story on the issue.[8]

Although there was spotty but regular national press coverage, the Richmond press covered DSIN activities closely. This was to be expected, since the Robins Company and the court were located in Richmond. All the television time allotted for Dalkon Shield news surrounding DSIN events went to DSIN because Robins's policy was to decline public comment.

Building the Collective Identity

Other nonprofit fundraisers we talked with were impressed by our 15% response rate from early DSIN mailings, but the rate was disappointing to DSIN leaders. We knew there were hundreds of thousands of affected women, most of them with absolutely no source of information. A major obstacle to our efforts was that the injured population was widely dispersed over the entire United States (as well as 101 other countries), which made group cohesion an enormous challenge. The geographical problem was exacerbated by DSIN's inability to contact most of these women directly.

Contacting the sheer numbers of persons involved in this case was daunting, even to the court. The bankruptcy court system generally interacts with several law firms who represent a bankrupt company or their creditors. The court was neither adequately funded nor constructed to communicate with hundreds of thousands of mass tort litigants. Early attempts by the other group and DSIN to gain access to the claimant mailing list had been initially stonewalled by the court and then made exceedingly difficult and expensive, as mentioned previously.

It has been noted by other observers of social movements that organized clienteles with a collective awareness of their constituencies present a serious threat to authority (Ruzek, 1978). Professionals and elites (in this case, the bankruptcy court officials and lawyers) are more likely to be challenged by clients like the Dalkon Shield survivors who, by becoming organized, can share some common values or expectations. "Fear of naming" is pervasive, and criticism of social and economic arrangements is very dangerous for those elites in control of major institutions (Fine, 1987).

The early task of building a community of Dalkon Shield survivors was tackled in three ways: (1) appealing to established organizations for help in locating other Dalkon Shield women, (2) channeling a massive amount of early energy and resources into a media campaign as a means to locate more women, and (3) creating local and regional chapters around the United States.

A Network of Local Chapters

Wilson (1973) has pointed out that sheer numbers make little difference in whether or not a collectivity should be treated as a social movement. The important question is what the potential scope of membership is thought to be. Apparently, the National Organization for Women exaggerated its membership numbers in its first year of existence (Davis, 1991).

We encouraged the perception that DSIN was a large organization by establishing a large number of regional affiliates, or chapters. Six women who attended the first Richmond rally agreed to form state chapters. Virtually every woman who contacted DSIN by phone or letter was asked to form a regional chapter. By the autumn of 1987 (within the first nine months of DSIN's existence), there were 13 chapters in 13 states. Eventually, there would be 18 chapters and 28 chapter coordinators. Unlike the women who founded NOW, DSIN leaders were not women who already had political savvy or connections; they just emerged among the women who volunteered.

Each chapter had a coordinator, who stayed in telephone contact with other members. In more rural or remote areas, there might be only a handful of women in communication with one another. In several urban areas, dozens or hundreds of women talked with one another. Most business was initiated and conducted by mail and telephone. In the end, there would be only one face-to-face meeting of 20 DSIN leaders—at the Richmond conference in February 1988. (See the section titled "First Appeals to Established Organizations" in Chapter 4 for a full account of this event.) Overall, there were few large public meetings, except in Bethlehem, Pennsylvania (DSIN's national office), Los Angeles, Dallas, and Denver. Some regional chapters had ongoing, small support groups who met regularly.

The chapter coordinators received an instruction packet on how to organize their chapter, frequent update mailings on the latest developments in the case, and telephone calls from the national leaders. The national office, which can be characterized as a kitchen-table operation, mailed voluminous amounts of material to the chapter coordinators, who could educate themselves and disseminate information to their local members and media contacts.

No real performance demands were placed on the chapter coordinators, and the degree of action and participation depended entirely on the chapter coordinator herself. It was a fairly risky strategy to induct totally unknown persons as spokespersons and leaders, but the top DSIN leaders felt that a structured set of guidelines about forming chapters and frequent phone calls would suffice as a starting point. These regional affiliates functioned basically as autonomous units. When women called the national office, they were referred to the regional chapters. This strategy was largely successful, both in terms of helping one another and of gaining legitimacy. It encouraged the perception that DSIN was a large organization more than a raw membership count would have done.

Over the first three years, chapter coordinators conducted a wide variety of activities in their local regions, some doing extensive and exhausting work on behalf of the organization, others serving primarily as telephone contacts for women in their area. Vera Davis, the Los Angeles coordinator, followed the original DSIN chapter instruction booklet to the letter and achieved an enormous degree of success in contacting and informing women in her area. She had at least one contact with a minimum of 5,000 women during her period of activism. She held regular meetings attended by hundreds of women.

Several DSIN leaders linked up with other consumer and health organizations in their home states. Vicki Pratt made numerous public appearances with consumer groups who were fighting product liability (or "tort") reform in Wisconsin. Sherry Fletcher also had working alliances with public interest and consumer organizations in Michigan. Jan Thompson worked with women's law organizations in Colorado. Cinders Murdock-Vaughan cooperated with the Resolve infertility group in Maryland. Donna Reeck and other western Pennsylvania women worked closely for two years with Lawyers for Consumer Rights, a consumer organization that was fighting the "tort reform" desired by big business. Reeck and I also testified in state legislative hearings on the issue. Reeck also worked intensively as the DSIN representative to a newly formed coalition group called International Victims of Corporate and Government Abuse (INVOCGA), which was composed of asbestos, Agent Orange, and Bhopal victims in addition to Dalkon Shield users.

DSIN's national officers were the hub for the chapters and all women who contacted the group. The three national officers were Cinders Murdock-Vaughan, Donna Reeck, and myself. All told, DSIN has had more than 20,000 direct contacts (telephone or letters) from people injured by the Dalkon Shield. Every media story would create a surge of calls.[9] Four people shared the national telephone support service and communicated regularly with one another. These contacts and the ongoing long-distance communications with the chapter leaders shaped the group's public action agenda.

WAGING THE FIGHT

DSIN activism did not commence with a superstructure or master plan. The *process* dictated the form and eventual structure of the group. We looked to allied organizations to build a base of support. With no prior experience, we sought advice and assistance from other social movements and women's health organizations, as well as making them our role models. Many groups were supportive but unable to advise us how to mount the challenge strategically. We learned as we went along, at every step.

Coincidentally, after the July 1987 Richmond rally, events in the bankruptcy litigation began to happen more rapidly than previously. The Rorer Company, another pharmaceutical firm, began negotiations to merge with Robins. The Dalkon Shield Claimants' Committee tried to file a separate lawsuit against three top-level Robins directors (Barrett, 1987). Judge Merhige found E. Claiborne Robins, Jr., in contempt of court for violating a court order concerning the recovery of illegal payments for prebankruptcy debts (Morris, 1987b).[10] The Dalkon Shield Claimants' Committee also tried but failed to have an emergency medical fund established for women incurring infertility treatment expenses (Morris, 1987a). The most critical events in the course of DSIN activism are discussed below.

November 1987—The Estimation of Total Claims

DSIN's limited energies and resources were directed to maintaining a presence in Richmond, both in the media and in the courtroom.

The group scheduled another major press conference at the YWCA in Richmond on November 5, 1987, to coincide with the three-day court hearing on the estimation of the total value of the Dalkon Shield claims.

We invited five other organizations to address the media. It was imperative to us then to invite international women's health groups in order to highlight the global impact of the case, which we had been discovering as women around the world began to learn of our work and to alarm us about their situation. (This is discussed in Chapter 2.) The six groups participating in the press conference were the International Health Network for Women, the Women's Global Network for Reproductive Rights, DSIN, the two other Dalkon Shield groups, and the National Women's Health Network.

Speakers at the press conference criticized the reorganization plan as fundamentally unfair to Dalkon Shield claimants and maximally beneficial to the Robins family and principal shareholders. Robins had been whining about its allegedly precarious financial situation in an attempt to minimize its obligations to Dalkon Shield victims; the focus at the conference was the fact that Robins was actually an extremely profitable company.

December 1987—DSIN *Criticizes the New Merger Plan*

DSIN held another press conference on December 17 at the National Press Club in Washington, D.C., to react to the most current version of the Robins reorganization plan, which was really about a merger of Robins with yet another pharmaceutical company that had recently entered the bidding war.

Under that version of the plan, Robins would have paid installments into the Trust over a seven-year period, funding them with junk bonds. This was unacceptable to DSIN members. The plan meant that Robins's shareholders would emerge from the bankruptcy court with the total value of their shares paid to them at the time of the final sale, and leave all the Dalkon Shield claimants waiting for compensation, based on whether or not there was enough real money in the Trust. DSIN speakers needed a simple, quick way to warn of this possibility and generated slogans at the press conference, such as:

"No easy payment plan for A. H. Robins!"
"While the lawyers battle it out in the courtroom, our lives hang
   in a statistical purgatory."

It seemed calculated to us that Robins issued a press release only a few hours before our press conference about the entry of a new bidder into the bidding war. (An almost identical event had upstaged a major press conference scheduled by another Dalkon Shield group in February 1987.) Although national press coverage was spotty for our press conference, the Richmond press sent their Washington correspondents and the event received wide coverage in Richmond and throughout Virginia. Women later sent us press clippings about the press conference from as far away as Toronto. A *Washington Post* article discussed the event. This was significant media coverage for the group.

February 1988—DSIN *Leaders Confer in Richmond*

There were so many new developments in the bankruptcy negotiations that all energies and resources went into publicly responding to them, instead of into trying to build a large membership base for the organization. In any case, there were no financial resources to do a large direct mailing.

DSIN national leaders decided to hold a conference of all DSIN leaders in Richmond to set DSIN's short-term priorities, to determine the major direction for DSIN's position on the anticipated reorganization plan, and to let the court know women were stepping up their demands. Eighteen women came from 13 different states for a two-day weekend conference on February 5 and 6, 1988. Our advance press releases suggested that DSIN's size was large by focusing on the number of states represented, not the number of women in attendance. Judge Merhige was invited to address the group, but he declined. He did offer us a tour of the new records center, which was coordinated by Michael Sheppard, then the bankruptcy court clerk. The conference sessions and press interviews were held again at the YWCA, where previous DSIN events had taken place.

The Richmond press coverage of the conference was significant. By fortunate coincidence, there had been a major breakthrough in the bankruptcy negotiations the day before the DSIN conference began. American Home Products reentered the bidding war for Robins, and the two companies announced a workable reorganization plan. The press was very interested in the claimants' reactions to the new developments. Women boldly criticized Robins, making local headlines in Richmond (Morris, 1988c). Also, a reporter from the *Wall Street Journal* was now tracking all our activities and attended our entire conference. He ultimately spent the weekend interacting with and interviewing all the women who attended (Barrett, 1988). In the end, Judge Merhige made a surprise appearance, addressing the group for about half an hour during our tour of the records center.

The Richmond conference was a milestone: It was the first opportunity for women in DSIN leadership roles to meet and to bond

with one another. Women who attended the conference gained from
it in ways that seemed personally therapeutic for them, and it provided an opportunity for their significant input into setting the priorities for the organization.

> In Richmond, I could look around me at a group of women who
> were *real*; we all had files there. It kind of brought it down for
> me and focused it. This is what it's all about. It's about women—
> women who have been denied reproductive freedom, since our
> existence on this planet, and we've had to suffer to this extent.
> (Victoria Pratt)

> I was able to voice my opinion [in Richmond]. I was able to get
> a load off my chest that I had not been able to do since 1972.
> When I went home, I got a good night's sleep that I had not
> gotten ever since I found out this thing had caused injuries in
> me. (Gloria Manago)

The meeting with the judge and the interest of the most important financial newspaper in the United States also validated the group's
efforts. A feature article on the conference and its significance to
overall events was eventually published in the *Wall Street Journal*
(Barrett, 1988).

March 1988—DSIN *Formally Objects to Robins's Plan*

At the Richmond conference, the other DSIN leaders authorized
me to prepare formal objections to the reorganization plan. The group
identified several issues of particular unfairness. I spent the next few
weeks researching and drafting DSIN's formal objections to the new
reorganization plan, based on the input from the women who had
attended the conference. Dr. Nadine Taub, law professor and director
of the Women's Rights Litigation Clinic at the Newhouse Center for
Law and Justice in Newark, New Jersey, coordinated and facilitated a
working session for me with several academic legal scholars, who
recommended the relevant and essential legal principles to address
in our objections. Later, I spoke and met with several more bankruptcy
and Dalkon Shield lawyers and then drafted a coherent, legally correct document for submission to the court, in accordance with standard legal procedure for a Chapter 11 proceeding.

Another precedent for DSIN came when I entered DSIN's objections
orally at the court hearing on objections to the plan, which was held
in March 1988. This meant official entry of at least some Dalkon

Shield women's voices into the court record, along with the other objections submitted by other lawyers. As anticipated by all parties, Judge Merhige affirmed the adequacy of the plan, and the official ballots for voting to approve or deny the plan were then mailed to all Robins's creditors, including the 197,000 Dalkon Shield claimants.[11]

May 1988—Dalkon Shield Groups Reject Plan

DSIN had had sporadic contact with other Dalkon Shield groups up to this point. One of the group's lawyer-advisors called on April 20, 1988, to suggest that the two groups form a coalition in opposition to the reorganization plan and that both groups publicly recommend that Dalkon Shield women should vote *no* to the proposed plan. Negotiating the speakers and agenda for this press conference was stressful and difficult. Extremely successful in the media, this press conference was another milestone in the life of DSIN. Coverage was very widespread in the national newspapers, including the major newspapers that carried this story continuously. (See Chapter 4 for a full discussion of this event and its meaning to DSIN.)

July 1988—The Confirmation Hearing

The results of the vote on the reorganization plan were not announced until the day of the confirmation hearing on the plan. All Robins Company shareholders and all Dalkon Shield claimants had the right, as prescribed by U.S. Bankruptcy Code, to vote on the plan (*In re* A. H. Robins Company, 1988). The plan was approved by an overwhelming majority of the Dalkon Shield claimants. Of the total group of 197,000 Dalkon Shield claimants, 141,094 mailed their ballots back to the court. Of these 141,094 claimants, 94.5% voted in favor of the plan. Only 7,884 claimants voted against the plan. More than 99% of the 19 million Robins common stockholders who voted also approved the plan (Morris, 1988a). With this resounding vote of confidence, Judge Merhige confirmed the plan at the confirmation hearing on July 19.

Lawyers from across the United States packed the courtroom for the highly charged confirmation hearing. The largest number of Dalkon Shield claimants at a court hearing to date also attended, due to the prehearing publicity conducted by DSIN to its members. During the hearing, Judge Merhige had an explosive exchange with Murray Drabkin, the lead Dalkon Shield Claimants' Committee lawyer. A newspaper account later revealed that the two men had been at odds over certain vital conditions of the plan right up to the last moment (Mintz, 1989c).

During a morning break at the hearing, Judge Merhige sent word to me through Mike Sheppard, his clerk, that I would not be allowed to address the court with my objections to the plan, as I had done in past hearings and was expecting to do again at this hearing. When the hearing resumed, I stood up anyway to address the court. Judge Merhige ordered me to sit down. Asserting my right to speak, I refused to sit. He had the federal marshals remove me from the courtroom.[12] During the stunned silence that followed this incident, about a dozen other women stood up and silently stormed out of the courtroom—and straight into a Richmond television camera on the courthouse steps to express our outrage for the unfair silencing of claimants' voices.

December 1988—DSIN Outrage over Firing of Trustees

After the Robins reorganization plan (to merge with American Home Products) was confirmed in July 1988, Judge Merhige approved the appointment of the five trustees for the Dalkon Shield Claimants' Trust Fund and urged them to begin setting up the Trust, despite the possibility of a long delay in starting payments should appeals of the plan be filed. These trustees function like a corporate board of directors. They receive an annuity, plus salary for each formal meeting, plus their expenses. They set the Trust's policies, approve all the employment decisions, and make decisions regarding all expenditures and investment strategies. Judge Merhige retains a supervisory role over all the budgets.

The selection of the five trustees had been a critical and heated political process during the long bankruptcy negotiations. Three of the five trustees were nominated by the Dalkon Shield Claimants' Committee, a compromise agreement against the judge's wishes (he wanted to place his own nominees in the majority). One of the trustees nominated by the Claimants' Committee was Ann Samani, a woman claimant who had been a member of the Claimants' Committee during the negotiations.

When the trustees began meeting on Trust business, Judge Merhige announced his displeasure with some of their early decisions, and he began to threaten, in the press, to fire some of them (Morris, 1988b). He ordered an investigation of them and held a hearing on the issues in October. The targets of the investigation turned out to be the three trustees nominated by the Claimants' Committee. DSIN members attended this explosive hearing, where Ann Samani, the Dalkon Shield claimant trustee, was treated particularly harshly by Judge Merhige from the bench. Mintz (1989c) described Merhige's behavior as highly irregular throughout the hearing. According to Mintz (1989c), Judge Merhige had acted as "a witness, a litigant, an advocate, and a judge of his own cause" at that hearing (p. 32). He gave his own testimony during the hearing and criticized the Dalkon Shield claimant trustee for being what he called "defiant of the court's authority." Merhige alleged that Samani had been rude to him in a trustee meeting during an exchange about the level of his continuing involvement in running the Trust. The other trustees testified that they did not see her question as defiant or rude (Mintz, 1989c).

Although DSIN was not privy to the behind-the-scenes politics, DSIN members who attended this hearing concluded from personal observations and commentary in the press that Judge Merhige was deeply invested in retaining a substantial amount of control over the Trust (Mintz, 1989c; Morris, 1988b).[13] We characterized this hearing as a "witch hunt." During this critical early stage of the Trust's development, Merhige used the court-ordered investigation of the trustees as a reason to freeze the trustees' access to the first monetary deposit into the Trust. The trustees had been deliberating over many banks, but Merhige insisted that a local Richmond bank be allowed to compete for the contract. In the end, Judge Merhige deposited the monies into a Richmond bank. During this time, Merhige appointed the bankruptcy court clerk, Mike Sheppard, as director of the Trust. No open search for the position was conducted.

By November, Merhige had fired the three trustees originally nominated by the Dalkon Shield Claimants' Committee, replacing two of them with his own original nominees. The fired trustees were accused of violating their fiduciary duty to the Trust (Labaton, 1988c). Merhige cited their slow progress in disbursing the funds and their resistance to close supervision by him. He accused them of "derelictions, open defiance of the court's authority, spending excessive time arguing and discussing ways to challenge the Court's supervisory role" (Mintz, 1989c, p. 33). Merhige also appointed the law firm of one of his former law clerks to be primary counsel to the Trust. By December 1989, Linda Thomason had been appointed as general counsel to the Trust. Previously, Thomason had worked in a Richmond law firm, where she had been part of the Robins defense team during the bankruptcy litigation.

For the first time in the whole bankruptcy proceedings, DSIN began to have frequent communications with Nancy Davis, one of the claimant members of the Claimants' Committee. Lawyers and claimants alike were appalled at this battle for control over the Trust. By this time, the work of the official Dalkon Shield Claimants' Committee was essentially over and its influence waning. DSIN held a press conference at the National Press Club, in conjunction with Nancy Davis, to express outrage at this turn of events, which many people believed threatened the integrity of the Trust. Unfortunately, this DSIN press conference was neither well attended nor widely reported.

SUMMARY

This chapter has reconstructed the events and issues that shaped DSIN's development from its beginnings as an information source for a repressed and submerged population, into a publicly identified and vocal movement waging a fight against a multinational corporation. What began as a relatively solitary information quest evolved into a nationwide political action group determined to protect the legal rights of millions of women. The inability to get full and reliable information about those rights forced the shift from pedagogy to politics. The social relations that developed within the movement are discussed in the next chapter.

4 The Complex Web of Relations

DSIN created a set of social relations where none had existed before. For almost 20 years, the vast majority of Dalkon Shield users had been isolated from one another. The emergence of DSIN into the public arena was an attempt to disrupt the culture of silence and to influence the official program of justice, which was controlled by corporate and legal elites. The net outcome of DSIN actions demonstrates that these women, who had little personal control over their individual contraceptive choices, were also relatively powerless to ameliorate the grave injustice they had experienced with this dangerous and unsafe birth control device. However, the chief contribution of DSIN may be that the victims were able to name the injustice publicly in their own voices, to advocate a notion of justice from their perspective, and to pressure the formal system to live up to its stated ideals.

This chapter treats the complex set of relations that evolved during the early stage of this social movement. Ten DSIN leaders contributed their perspectives to these topics by participating in structured interviews.

INTERNAL DSIN RELATIONS

There were varying types of relations among the people who became part of DSIN. Some women sent donations and were content to receive the newsletter or to make an occasional telephone call to the DSIN hotline with a personal concern. Chapter coordinators had both the energy and personal resources to implement the DSIN agenda of information and empowerment. Some chapter coordinators maintained direct contact with one another. Finally, the top four to six leaders stayed in frequent communication with one another and directed the public, political agenda.

I was the sole founder, president, and spokesperson for DSIN in the first few months. My chief advisors were my husband, who had worked in a grass-roots environmental group, and Sybil Shainwald, a former president of the National Women's Health Network board of directors. Shainwald introduced me (by telephone) to Sherry Fletcher, a Dalkon Shield woman in Michigan who was eager to work on this with me. Fletcher and I began to network with established organizations. We made the earliest attempts to gain allies and seek funding sources, as well as buoy each other's spirits to push on with the "good fight" in the first few months. As time went on, Cinders Murdock-Vaughan and Donna Reeck became DSIN officers (vice-president and secretary, respectively). The three of us were DSIN's national spokespersons. We were on the telephone constantly with one another and the chapter leaders. Input from chapter coordinators always helped frame the agenda as events and process unfolded.

When we first began to implement public protest actions, we were not aware of the complexity of this issue. Murdock-Vaughan reflected on how much we learned *after* we had completed the first Richmond rally. It was a theme that continued throughout the three years of intense participation: "We were amazed by what we had accomplished at that rally, but awed by all the agendas out there, all the people with vested interests who were hanging around in the back of the room" (Cinders Murdock-Vaughan). Other DSIN leaders felt the same way once they became involved and participated in DSIN-sponsored events:

> It was so overwhelming to learn how many levels there were. It wasn't just a simple case of somebody did something wrong and they should be held accountable for it. There was all this politics and power trips going on, too. That was sort of upsetting, realizing the complexity of it. (Jan Thompson)

ALLIES AND ALLIANCES

First Appeals to Established Organizations

DSIN members had spent the months before the July 1987 Richmond rally talking on the telephone to other national organizations, trying to gain endorsements for this neophyte organization and the Richmond rally. Gaining allies was an important strategy for us, because we needed advice on organizing strategies and affirmation of our efforts. Support and endorsement from existing groups would help

DSIN project itself as a large pressure group, belying its small membership at that time. DSIN members began contacting at least 30 different national organizations for support.

Additionally, during four Richmond rally planning trips in the spring of 1987, Murdock-Vaughan and I met with and spoke with representatives of 20 Richmond area community organizations. We expected that the seven local Richmond women's and reproductive rights groups, as well as local individuals recommended to us, would be willing allies. The president of the local NOW chapter and the head of a state-wide women's legal organization were receptive but, to our surprise, the other feminist groups declined involvement, saying either that this issue was not relevant to their own organizational missions or that their groups were already overcommitted to other projects. We were never able to meet these women in person.

DSIN's strongest Richmond allies came from the local human rights groups, mostly from women of color who were members of the local Richmond Black Women's Political Network and other member groups of the Richmond Human Rights Coalition. Additional supporters were the local Common Cause branch, the local peace and justice organization, the Richmond branch of the Women's International League for Peace and Freedom, the Richmond YWCA,[1] and several professors at Virginia Commonwealth University, including Diana Scully, a sociology professor who has written about medical sexism (1980, in press). Ultimately, 14 national and Richmond organizations agreed to officially sponsor the first event.

The success of that rally, in terms of numbers of participants, however, came from the mobilization of African-American women in the Richmond area. Murdock-Vaughan and I found these women to be most receptive to us. They invited us into their homes and opened their hearts to us readily in the months preceding the rally. They spoke movingly about their own experiences with medical abuse, and they knew Dalkon Shield women in their community who had suffered as we had. Many of the women of color who turned out in force for the first rally did so partly on behalf of women they knew in Richmond who could not afford to be public in this manner. In fact, it was difficult for us to convince Dalkon Shield women living in Richmond to come out publicly during the years of our activism there. The women who contacted us told us they felt too vulnerable. Fran Cleary, the Richmond chapter leader, was an exception. Throughout most of DSIN activism in Richmond, she was the only Richmond Dalkon Shield survivor who participated publicly.

The Women's Health Movement Organizations

With limited avenues for direct contact with other victims and no previous organizing experience, DSIN turned to well-known women's health movement organizations for help in locating women, for gaining moral support and validation that our work was important, and for advice about grass-roots organizing. When DSIN leaders began organizing in 1987, we were naive about being publicly political. We pursued role models from feminist organizations, assuming that these women could and would help us learn quickly.

The two most prominent national feminist women's health rights organizations (National Women's Health Network and Boston Women's Health Book Collective) seemed to be natural allies, since these groups had been founded by women who had written critiques of the sexist medical care system and had debated the politics of women's health in many public forums. When I entered the Dalkon Shield "scene" in 1987, the women's health movement already had a history of being vocal and, in addition to lawyers who litigated cases, women's health leaders had acted as primary advocates on behalf of Dalkon Shield users. A significant outcome of the women's health movement in the 1970s was the reassessment of the hazards of contraceptive drugs and devices: "Feminists have waged major battles against powerful drug interests to combat the wave of iatrogenic disease that experts ignored or denied" (Ruzek, 1978, p. 226). Based on this history, we presumed that we could establish an open, easy rapport with these established groups. That did not happen, however.

My own interactions with the National Women's Health Network (NWHN) began in 1986, as a result of contacting Sybil Shainwald, a NWHN board member at that time. I first contacted her when I saw an article on the Shield in the NWHN newsletter. She encouraged me to pursue my own idea, which was to recommend the creation of a subcommittee on the Dalkon Shield within NWHN. (This predated the creation of DSIN.) I made several attempts to bring that proposal to NWHN, but I did not receive support from the group's executive director in Washington, D.C. (See the section entitled "Seeking Support and Assistance" in Chapter 3 for a discussion of the attempt.) I do not know why my appeals went unanswered. After DSIN was formed, I did receive some early letters of support from Judy Norsigian, a Boston Women's Health Book Collective (BWHBC) leader. She promised several times to put us in touch with other women's health groups and to make some press contacts for us (Norsigian, personal communications, 1987), but never did. Ultimately, none of the contacts DSIN made in these areas came via BWHBC.

There were two main reasons for our difficulties in gaining their cooperation on this issue. The first reason involved the context of reproductive rights politics in 1987–1988. Some women's health movement leaders began supporting the reintroduction of IUDs and newer high-tech contraceptive methods, during this period when reproductive rights were again being threatened and restricted. This was also the direction of the general women's movement—to offer women more "choice" by supporting high-tech contraceptive methods then in development, for example, the Norplant implant and the Depo Provera injectable.[2]

A short time after DSIN was created in 1987, two developments influenced the politics of contraception in the United States. Feminist media writers were beginning to raise public awareness of RU-486, the new contragestive drug developed in France as an alternative to conventional abortion. RU-486 seemed, to feminists, to be a solution to the political pressures being exerted by anti-choice forces, since this pill purportedly would give women more personal control and privacy regarding their reproductive decisions (Fraser, 1988; Sweet, 1988). Also, feminist health groups were feeling pressure from population control agencies, which believed they were an obstacle to expanding contraceptive options. Population control groups now blamed the Dalkon Shield settlement for reducing research and development on new contraceptives, out of liability fears. Comments by Norsigian and Swenson, BWHBC leaders, suggest the dilemmas facing feminist health activists with regard to new contraceptive developments.

> Even Norma Swenson of the Boston Women's Health Book Collective, who emphasizes that the Dalkon Shield settlement represents a hard-fought victory for the women's health movement, admits that it had the ironic by-product of "chilling manufacturers." (Fraser, 1988, p. 44)

Then, the new Paragard IUD hit the market in May 1988 (Fraser, 1988; Lang, 1988). We began to read and see on television indications that NWHN leaders supported the reintroduction of IUDs. First, Adriane Fugh-Berman, a NWHN board member appearing as a panelist on a February 1989 segment of the television show "Nightline" on new birth control methods, recommended a more widespread adoption of IUDs and made reference to "frivolous" IUD lawsuits. A ques-

tion from the show's commentator prompted her to clarify that she did not mean to imply that the Dalkon Shield lawsuits were frivolous, which leaves her meaning completely unclear. After discussing this with other DSIN leaders, I sent a letter of protest to NWHN. No one from NWHN ever responded to my letter. I was disappointed at the lack of dialogue or debate on this issue. My interpretation was that victims' voices were being silenced.

Second, a NWHN fundraising appeal indicates that, around the same time, the group was taking credit for the establishment of better-informed consent procedures for IUD use—another sign of their approval of IUDs.

> Our accomplishments—better informed consent with IUDs, an upcoming hearing on experimental condoms and a new federal breast cancer prevention study—show that if the Network assiduously attempts to change health policies, the Network makes changes. (Rennie, NWHN memo, February 28, 1989)

Third, NWHN distributed a written packet of information on IUDs, as they do on many topics concerning women's health issues. This pamphlet supported the use of IUDs. The pamphlet contained the sentence: "We also advise that women using the IUD be over thirty years old and have no interest in bearing any more children" (NWHN pamphlet, 1986). Although the pamphlet discussed pelvic inflammatory disease (PID) in the next paragraph, it did not elucidate the connection between PID and the advice to the women over 30. Surely this lack of explanation bordered on misinformation: It is not acceptable for anyone, including women over 30 with no childbearing plans, to risk contracting PID.

DSIN was opposed to any type of support for the reintroduction of IUDs because we had received correspondence and telephone calls from women injured by other types of IUDs. DSIN files contain records of women injured by the Cu-7 (Copper 7), the Saf-T-Coil, Lippes Loop, the Shamrock, and other types of IUDs that women could not even identify correctly. The injuries described were identical to Shield injuries. When these women read or saw press stories on the Shield, they started calling DSIN for help—there was nowhere else for them to turn.

Due to this increasing contact with other IUD users, DSIN started an IUD registry of sorts with first-person accounts, unsolicited medical records, and women's hand-drawn pictures of IUDs that we did not even recognize. DSIN leaders concluded from the severity of the injuries and the similarity of mistreatment among these women that safety issues related to IUDs are unresolved and that the medical literature is contradictory. Furthermore, articles have been published that allege corporate misbehavior, similar to that of Robins, on the part of G. D. Searle & Co., manufacturer of the Copper 7 IUD (Glaberson, 1985; Mintz, 1988, 1989a). These circumstances were the basis for our skepticism about any enthusiasm for new IUD models. We determined from these contacts that a long-term goal of DSIN might be to expand the group to include women with injuries from all IUDs. We began networking and communicating regularly with women injured by other IUDs.

As we experienced it in the later 1980s, Shainwald was the only NWHN leader maintaining a strong public stand against the Dalkon Shield and other IUDs, while other NWHN board members' actions and rhetoric diverged. The long history of this case followed two waves of activity: In the early 1970s, feminist health activists championed the issue, joining doctors and other public health advocates in demanding that the device be removed from the market. Then, in the mid-1980s, Dalkon Shield women themselves emerged to continue the fight when the Robins Company sought bankruptcy protection in order to avoid its responsibility to the injured women. Ironically, many women activists in the early women's health movement realized the dangers of the Dalkon Shield before Dalkon Shield users themselves got this information. DSIN's rise was a response partly to the inability of Dalkon Shield users to get the level of cooperation they desired from existing women's health groups. The lack of support for our needs precipitated the evolution of DSIN as a "single-issue" organization.

Many Dalkon Shield women were also unsettled by what we perceived to be vacillation and inconsistency in the women's health movement's original commitment to stricter government testing, regulation, and surveillance of new drugs and medical devices. Several other developments perplexed us. In 1988, a NWHN fundraising appeal contained the following statement: "The Network is committed to ensuring that all drugs and devices for women are proven safe and effective *before* they are approved" (National Women's Health Network, memo, August 25, 1988). However, around the same time, I read that both NWHN and BWHBC were giving early support for RU-486, which was quite a new technology at that time. NWHN and BWHBC spokespersons were quoted in the press as approving the entry of RU-486 into the United States, even on the black market, if necessary:

> At the Boston Women's Health Book Collective, Norma Swenson argues
> that RU-486 would save so many women around the world from death
> by botched abortion that it would be worth it for women's groups to
> organize its underground use. (Fraser, 1988, p. 44)

Many DSIN leaders who followed contraceptive developments were
alarmed at the danger that this new and relatively unknown drug
would be unsupervised and misused. We feared great harm to women's
bodies.[3]

Also in 1988, NWHN accepted $10,000 from Procter & Gamble to
sponsor a conference on women's health. This seemed, to me, a startling shift of NWHN founding policy not to accept corporate money,
particularly from companies with ties to the pharmaceutical industry. (Procter & Gamble subsidiaries include the Richardson-Vicks and
G. D. Searle's over-the-counter pharmaceutical firms.) Minutes of
NWHN's November 1988 board meeting may explain the rationale for
accepting this corporate money:

> The question is whether with our 1989 projected deficit if [*sic*]
> we want to direct our staff to seek corporate money. Decision:
> We direct our staff to seek corporate money under guidelines to
> be set by the board. Decision: The following statement will update
> our decision regarding corporate fundraising from 10 years ago.
> Decision: We do not want to take money from corporations
> linked with: tobacco, porn, or alcohol.

These developments in the women's health movement organizations were disillusioning. I—and other early DSIN leaders—felt aban-
doned at a critical moment of need, when the urgency of the A. H.
Robins bankruptcy proceedings presented an opportunity to apply
renewed pressure for social change in medical practice and pharmaceutical company conduct.

The grandest disappointment to us came with the announcement
of a new group called the Reproductive Health Technologies Project.
This organization was created in 1988 to promote public education
on RU-486 and to counter the anti-choice organizations. Advisors to
this project included: Population Council, Population Crisis Committee, American College of Obstetrics and Gynecology, Planned Parenthood USA, Women's Legal Defense Fund, National Women's Health
Network, Boston Women's Health Book Collective, National Abortion
Rights Action League, Federation of Feminist Women's Health Cen-
tres, and National Black Women's Health Project ("Groups in USA

. . . ," 1989). It seemed to us that the willingness of women's health movement leaders to cooperate with the patriarchal institutions of power was a strategy to make them appear neutral about new contraceptive technologies. Why did they seem willing to mute their historical adversarial stance? Their rhetoric about the long-term effects and safety of drugs and their approval of potent pharmaceutical products were a glaring contradiction.

Norsigian (1992) laments the development of single-issue groups within the women's health movement: "In times of diminishing resources, it is difficult to keep up the networking and coalition-building. Also, the emergence of 'single-issue' organizations may make it harder to keep the broader feminist context in focus" (p. 12).

Given our experience, I am at a loss to define the "broader feminist context." Although NWHN's purpose is to champion and reform women's health care, it seems to do so at a distance from most women. The lack of coordination between NWHN and victims/survivors of medical abuse or women interested in general health issues is unfortunate and disappointing.

DSIN is not the only single-issue women's health group. DES Action is a nationwide organization that has had great success advocating for DES victims for more than 17 years. The Hysterectomy Education and Resource Services (HERS) group is another example of grass-roots organizing by women enraged by the alarmingly high rates of surgical and medical abuse. There are also breast cancer groups, the Endometriosis Association, and several cesarean prevention organizations. The silicone gel breast implant victims currently operate in an uncoordinated collection of support groups, according to a woman who hopes to inspire greater cohesion of these women (N. Fluir, personal communication, September 23, 1992).

I believe that most of these organizations arose primarily out of some women's passionate concern for assisting and supporting other women in similar circumstances. From personal communications with the founders of DES Action and HERS, I know this to be the case with at least those two groups. Some—not all—of these groups' founders would label themselves feminists.

The second reason for the lack of cooperation that we desired from NWHN and BWHBC was the factionalism and power struggles within women's health movement organizations at the time DSIN emerged. In 1986–1987, the election process for NWHN's board of directors was marred by internal struggles. As a NWHN member and candidate, I received a series of letters from prominent women's health activists who criticized both the tampering with the election process and the character assassination (P. Chesler, personal communication, 1986; M. Harrison, personal communication, 1986). It may also be that the distraction of internal politics seriously hindered NWHN's ability to lend assistance when we most urgently needed it.

Some women- and feminist-identified health groups did offer open and unqualified support to DSIN. Frequent interactions and a positive working relationship were maintained with the Women's Global Network for Reproductive Rights, based in the Netherlands. Also, some individual U.S. health centers supported DSIN enthusiastically, including the Santa Cruz Women's Health Collective, the New Hampshire Feminist Health Collective, and the Elizabeth Blackwell Health Center in Philadelphia. As mentioned previously, our contacts with infertility organizations were strong. Resolve, Inc., and other infertility support organizations communicated regularly with DSIN. Thus, although the so-called women's health movement did not offer DSIN much support and advice, we had regional and international contact with individual feminist women's health organizations.

In the final analysis, the relationship between Dalkon Shield activists and the U.S. women's health movement leaders has, unfortunately, been marginal. I would characterize our relations as distant, strained, and infrequent. This pattern is not unique to DSIN:

> It is disappointing, however, to recognize that while feminists, by definition, are in conflict with men in a patriarchal society, we are also in internal conflict within our own feminist organizations because of our differences. (MacPherson, 1986, p. 55)

In any event, I regret that our differences were not worked out through dialogue with one another; instead, there has been mostly avoidance by all parties.

The Women's Movement Organizations

After the attempt to gain support from the women's health organizations, DSIN leaders began to network with known women political activists and the feminist press. Because these activist women were also role models for waging a fight against the patriarchal institutions of power, we then diverted energy to appealing to these groups for support. Early contacts with NOW were positive. Staff members recommended organizing strategies and reported DSIN news in their national newspaper, the *NOW Times*. The Women's Legal Defense Fund declined active involvement in our legal battles, citing other priorities and the lack of legal specialists to tackle this complex bankruptcy litigation. However, they did express sympathy and encouragement. Dr. Nadine Taub, director of the Rutgers-based Women's Rights Litigation Clinic, contacted feminist writers and the press for DSIN,[4] convened an important working session with other legal scholars on legal principles related to DSIN opposition to the reorganization plan, and was continuously available with advice on political strategy. Ruth Mandel, director of the Center for the American Woman in Politics at the Eagleton Institute of Rutgers University, also lent moral support and networking assistance to DSIN.

The Challenge to "Choice." By the time of the Robins bankruptcy in 1987, the political pressures mentioned previously had created new demands on all women's movement organizations as a result of the renewed threat to reproductive rights. The politics of choice began to usurp the safety issues involved in birth control again. For Dalkon Shield activists, this timing was unfortunate.

The bankruptcy proceedings against A. H. Robins coincided with the historical moment when RU-486 was beginning to receive publicity in the United States. After articles by feminist writers appeared in the press, a rash of articles by anti-choice movement leaders about RU-486 also began to appear. One element of their criticism of RU-486 involved drawing parallels to the Dalkon Shield, from the standpoint of RU-486's newness and the lack of information on its long-term safety (Allen, 1989). These groups also attacked the reintroduction of IUDs because of their abortifacient properties.[5] Anti-choice groups began using the Dalkon Shield example as a reason to block new birth control developments completely.

I experienced these new political dilemmas personally when I was invited to participate on a "Birth Control Technologies" panel at the 1988 NOW convention in Buffalo. Lisa Kaeser, from the Alan Guttmacher Institute (a prominent family-planning agency), was also on the panel. She spoke about the urgent need for more contraceptive options. She profiled high-tech methods that were considered promising at that time—the Norplant implant, RU-486, the vaginal ring, and Depo Provera. Although I found the panel's attendees sympathetic to my account of the Dalkon Shield tragedy and the need for continuing vigilance on contraceptive safety issues, I was dismayed by what happened at a later session. The convention planks on reproductive rights called for increased research and development of the new high-tech contraceptive methods that Kaeser had spoken of on the panel as the way to protect "choice." In my opinion, contraceptive safety issues were again submerged by the current political climate threatening the choice issue. Many feminists who had assailed the pharmaceutical industry about the Dalkon Shield in the 1970s were now at a different level of thinking on the whole issue relative to Dalkon Shield women, who were just now uniting and actively fighting the Robins Company.

The top DSIN leadership was pro-choice on reproductive rights, which was an important factor in the search for allies. I identified myself as a feminist. Although chapter leaders and members felt bonded because of their similar injuries from the Dalkon Shield, there were both pro-choice and anti-choice women in DSIN. Some DSIN chapter leaders who identified themselves as "right-to-lifers" encouraged the DSIN national officers to contact anti-choice groups, such as Concerned Women of America, for support. DSIN appealed to many groups for moral and financial support, but any alliance or even any overture to anti-choice groups was philosophically and politically unacceptable to DSIN's national leadership. The national leaders consciously avoided association with anti-choice groups. However, as I experienced it, pro-choice groups isolated the Dalkon Shield cause out of fear that drawing parallels to the Shield would further restrict abortion and the development of new contraceptive choices.

Many women who engage in social activism, even on so-called women's issues such as the Dalkon Shield, do not consider themselves feminists, even if their actions, philosophy, and behavior fit the profile of feminism. Many Dalkon Shield women activists were motivated to action primarily by their passion to protect women's rights *to be able* to reproduce. By contrast, the organized feminist movement has concentrated all its resources and energies into fighting for women's rights *not* to be obliged to reproduce. Protecting the right to motherhood presents a conflict for the organized feminist movement at large. This had previously created a rift between white feminists and women of color, whose exposure to sterilization abuse was increased as a consequence of feminist contraceptive battles (Ruzek, 1978).

Fighting for the right to prevent pregnancy and fighting to protect the right to motherhood should not be mutually exclusive goals for the feminist community. The political realities involving battles over choice have led the feminist movement to see motherhood as a for-it or against-it choice. Women who do not identify themselves as feminists nevertheless can—and do—understand gender inequality and fight against abuses of male power. Their failure to identify with the feminist movement and invoke it to explain their own political behaviors often arises because the startling lack of support for motherhood on the part of the organized feminist movement is so profound that it seems like a stance *against* motherhood. This issue is a significant point of divergence for women who see both rights as vital.

Public Interest and Consumer Organizations

DSIN received the most acceptance and support from other victims' and human rights organizations, as well as public interest legal and health groups. The closest allies and friends of DSIN emerged from the consumer and public interest organizations that were deeply engaged in battles over product liability and other instances of corporate abuse of the public trust. In 1987, the Civil Justice Foundation made two modest grants to DSIN. Later, Lawyers for Consumer Rights (LCR), a non-profit consumer rights group in Pennsylvania (now defunct), gave modest financial assistance in the form of covering printing and mailing costs for several issues of the DSIN newsletter. LCR reported Dalkon Shield developments and DSIN activity in its own publications, invited DSIN to participate with other groups as a coalition at press conferences around Pennsylvania, and gave substantial moral support, principally from Barbara DeVane, LCR's executive director. Charlie Inlander, president of the People's Medical Society, a national, consumer-oriented health organization based in Allentown, Pennsylvania, also gave much encouragement and advice.

As a result of our networking with other organizations, we were invited to participate in events they sponsored. Several chapter leaders in Pennsylvania attended multiple press conferences around the state dealing with product liability and tort reform. Reeck and I both testified at Pennsylvania legislative hearings. Murdock-Vaughan represented DSIN at several events sponsored by Ralph Nader in the Washington, DC, area. Vicki Pratt, DSIN's Wisconsin chapter leader, attended training conferences for activist leaders and has joined other consumer groups in lobbying against tort reform. DSIN participated actively at a New York conference in 1987 sponsored by a global organization called Health Action International, which is linked to the International Organization of Consumer Unions. Through this connection, we met the leaders of other single-issue organizations. Our commonality was victimization from corporate abuse. With these groups, DSIN became a founding member of a new organization called the International Network of Victims of Corporate and Government Abuse (INVOGGA); DSIN member Donna Reeck worked intensively with this group. Other INVOGGA member groups organized survivors of Agent Orange, Bhopal, and asbestos.

In April 1991, DSIN participated in a People's Tribunal on Industrial Hazards and Human Rights at Yale Law School. The tribunal, with permanent offices in Italy, organizes events around the globe on various human rights themes. Representatives of about a dozen victims' groups offered testimony during a three-day hearing to a panel of international judges, which later issued a finding of gross violations of fundamental human rights perpetrated by corporations and government agencies. It was profoundly moving and a great privilege to meet with and hear people from all over the globe who have been abused, mistreated, and even scorned in ways that are similar to the Dalkon Shield case. Reeck also represented DSIN and gave a moving speech to thunderous applause at the street theater event in New York City called "Earth Day–Wall Street Action" in 1990. The goal of this event, sponsored by more than 50 environmental and radical political groups, was to close the New York Stock Exchange for a day in order to focus attention on environmental degradation due to corporate greed (Lorch, 1990, p. B5).

Relationships with these groups, none of which were gender-specific, were congenial and without conflict or tension. In fact, these relations probably helped DSIN by transcending the gender-identified nature of the issue. In this way, more allies were engaged in our own cause. We felt more like peers in our relations with these groups—much more so than in our relations with the women's health movement organizations. There are several possible explanations for this: (1) Perhaps the commonalities of our shared victimizations gave rise to our camaraderie; (2) we were all single-issue organizations with clearly different constituencies that did not overlap; and (3) we were all poor financially, and the causes we championed were not popular with mainstream foundations; therefore, we were not competing with one another for resources.

OTHER DALKON SHIELD ORGANIZATIONS

In addition to DSIN, there were three other organized groups of Dalkon Shield women: two U.S. groups (referred to herein as Group A and Group B) and Dalkon Shield Action Canada (DSAC), with chapters in Montreal, Toronto, and Vancouver. DSIN members discovered the existence of these other groups after we began publishing the DSIN newsletter in January 1987. The social relations among all the groups are discussed here in terms of issues of coalition building, conflict, conflict resolution, and fragmentation among the groups.

DSIN had no ongoing relations with Group A during the bankruptcy proceedings. There are two reasons for this. First, the sole content of my first outreach telephone call to the group—with a woman who was also a Dalkon Shield claimant and the group's director—was about whether or not I wanted a referral to a lawyer to represent my case. I concluded from that conversation that this group was a lawyer-referral service and, therefore, did not have a mission compatible with that of DSIN. Later we received printed matter from a lawyer who referred to himself as Group A's "counsel." From my perspective, this was an unacceptable relationship for a legitimate, nonprofit support organization.

The second reason for not pursuing an alliance with Group A was the negative confrontation in Richmond between three DSIN and DSAC leaders and a lawyer prominently associated with Group A. This appalling episode destroyed our desire for a continuing relationship with this group. The details of this event are treated in the next section, entitled "Conflicts and Confrontations."

Group B first reached out to DSIN in the first months of our existence. I received a detailed set of documents, on impressive-looking official stationery, that included an honorable and complex organizational charter and mission statement as well as a description of an impressive board of directors. DSIN did not have a comparable portfolio. The group's stated purposes included providing information on the case, assisting women in locating infertility help, promoting research into PID, developing guidelines for marketing and testing new drugs, and promoting corporate responsibility.

DSIN's early relations with Group B were reserved and cautious. The skepticism that we felt toward Group B arose principally because the group's lawyer/advisor was so prominent in conducting the group's business. Group B's early press releases listed him and his secretary as the primary contact persons. Many of my earliest phone conversations were with this man—not the women organizers. He also offended me by suggesting then that DSIN fold into Group B and that I become the East Coast spokesperson for Group B.

Murdock-Vaughan and I were invited by the women to visit Group B in August 1987 to discuss the prospects of a coalition. On that trip, I discovered that the group's mailing address and primary business site were this lawyer's office. We found the women sincere about and committed to supporting other Dalkon Shield women, but the trip only confirmed my early doubts about this lawyer's intense participation. There was a cordial interaction between the women in both groups, but I was resistant to any coalition plan.

Conflicts and Confrontations

In November 1987, DSIN invited Group B to participate in a Richmond press conference, which DSIN organized for the court hearing on the total value of the Dalkon Shield claims. The group's chairwoman did participate in the press conference. Interaction was cordial but reserved.

The women leaders of Group A and Group B were interested in meeting with DSIN leaders on the day of the November 1987 press conference in Richmond. Both women articulated a desire to explore mutual future projects with DSIN and DSAC. Nora Morin (from Montreal), Murdock-Vaughan, and I agreed to meet with them. However, we were alarmed that six male lawyers accompanied the women from Groups A and B to this meeting. Because the invitation for a meeting had come from the women and concerned the victims' organizations, Morin, Murdock-Vaughan, and I refused to talk to these women until the lawyers left. The lawyers retreated to another section of the restaurant for the interim.

Both women raised the prospect of a working coalition of the four groups. Murdock-Vaughan and I again expressed skepticism of the intensive lawyer participation in their groups, which was reinforced by the presence of so many lawyers at this very meeting. This skepticism emanated from our fear that these lawyers sought control of the women's groups in order to facilitate their own financial goals. At this time, we were still figuring out who the players were, what their agendas were, and whose interests were compatible with ours: "We spent days processing an hour-long meeting, trying to figure out who had the hidden agenda" (Cinders Murdock-Vaughan).

The lawyers returned a short time later and asked to join the discussion. In their absence, there had been no real progress in forming a coalition. The lawyer who described himself in his written literature as counsel to Group A then accused us, in what we perceived as a hostile tone, of practicing law without a license, and he made what we heard as an implied threat that we would face "sanctions" if we continued our activities. The lawyer for Group B stood by and said nothing. We felt as if we had been intimidated; we rebuffed them and left abruptly. DSIN made no further attempts to communicate with Group A after this incident.

This episode heightened our sense of victimization. We were now fearful that the conjunction of corporate interests extended beyond the infamous Robins Company and Aetna, its insurer. We began to see at least five ways that Dalkon Shield women could experience victimization: (1) by the pharmaceutical industry, which had callously created the device that caused the damages; (2) by the insurance industry, which was concerned to minimize damage awards; (3) by doctors who were more interested in protecting themselves against liability claims than in helping women heal or attain compensation, or both; (4) by lawyers, like this one, who treated us in a manner that we could only perceive as intimidating; and (5) by the court system, which seemed to us to be more deferential to the Robins Company interests.

Over the next two years, we perceived both Group A and Group B to be advancing lawyers' goals. We determined to proceed with our own agenda rather than to spend our scant resources working through painful coalition negotiations with these two groups.

We did not experience the same problems or reservations with DSAC, the women-centered Canadian group. There was a much more equitable exchange of information and collaboration between DSIN and DSAC.

Uneasy Coalition

The issue of the vote on the reorganization plan was a critical political moment for all the Dalkon Shield groups. DSIN was empowering some women by providing them information so they could at least monitor the bankruptcy negotiations and learn how to protect their own compensation claims. DSIN leaders hoped that empowered women could make a difference in the outcome of the vote on any plan in such a way as to place the interests of the Dalkon Shield claimants— and not those of the Robins shareholders—foremost. (Ultimately, however, DSIN was never able to contact more than a tiny percentage of the total number of claimants and was unable to affect the vote significantly.)

The idea of getting revenge against Robins simmered underneath DSIN's public agenda from the beginning of the group's activism. Many women, on their first contact with DSIN, suggested plans for initiating a boycott against A. H. Robins profitable over-the-counter products. However, as both the case and DSIN evolved through time, certain realities of the situation tempered this possibility. First, we were unable to afford the cost of the mailing list of claimants, as mentioned in Chapter 3, and were thereby prevented from contacting the vast majority of claimants directly; second, the negotiations were happening so fast that even a massive media strategy to locate and inform claimants about the unfair features of the plan would not have been possible (given our limited resources); and finally, most of the women we were in contact with were counting on financial compensation of some kind and could not support jeopardizing the final plan.

> One of the things that we always saw but most women didn't and *still* don't . . . most women had an inflated notion of how much money they were going to get, and we feared that they wouldn't recognize the injustice until they received the paltry amount that they were going to get. That was information that we were hard-pressed to share with women. We often jostled over money as justice. (Cinders Murdock-Vaughan)

About six months later, Group B suggested a joint press conference with DSIN to express opposition to the reorganization plan. Group B's lawyer/advisor called on April 20, 1988, to suggest what he called a "coalition" press conference. Coincidentally, at this time DSIN was networking with and beginning to gain allies within the national women's rights organizations in Washington, DC. We had begun to receive advice and assistance from Kathy Bonk, a feminist activist and skilled media specialist well known within the women's movement.

At the time of this press conference invitation, Bonk was coordinating introductions for DSIN to potential fundraising experts, and she was giving DSIN invaluable free advice on organizational growth and development. I sought Bonk's advice about whether DSIN should participate in the proposed press conference, and she made an instantaneous offer to coordinate it with all her resources—staff, facilities, her own time, written materials, and press contacts. It was a magnanimous gesture.

The process of planning this event was significant in the life of DSIN. Up to this point, DSIN had initiated all press conferences in Richmond in connection with critical developments in the bankruptcy litigation. Now, DSIN was the invitee. The two groups would have to negotiate who the speakers and what the content of the event would be. The earlier sense of suspicion and skepticism on my part was reinforced by the fact that the lawyer—not the women leaders—had extended the invitation to us and handled all the negotiations about the details.

In April 1988, DSIN's national office conducted a telephone poll of chapter leaders in order to determine DSIN's position on the plan: Should we approve it or recommend its rejection? Six leaders voted for a moderate DSIN position on the plan, which meant that we should demand modifications to the existing reorganization plan. Four oth-

ers voted to sack the entire plan, if necessary, to demonstrate a commitment to bringing all responsible parties to full accountability. One
chapter leader abstained from the vote. Additionally, the majority of
telephone contacts with other DSIN members during this period
showed a clear preference for modification, not destruction, of the
plan.

I believed that a position on this issue that was unpopular with
other Dalkon Shield women would have reduced DSIN, in the public
eye, to a radical fringe group—a negative development from my perspective. Murdock-Vaughan felt strongly that DSIN should boldly urge
rejection of the reorganization plan, based on the continuing injustice inherent in it. Unfairnesses in the plan included (1) immunity to
all third parties from any further prosecutions, (2) shareholders' privi-
leged status in the plan, and (3) unfair weighting of the vote on the
plan. "It was a matter of principle and not reality . . . we knew there
was little chance of actually winning, but it was important to protest
the unfairness of this plan, nevertheless" (Cinders Murdock-Vaughan).
The close vote and the difference of opinion among top Dalkon Shield
leaders signaled a critical moment for the organization.

In spite of the close call, I took this voice vote as a mandate from
the chapter leaders to shape DSIN's future public action agenda in favor
of modification, not destruction, of the plan. A face-to-face meeting
on this issue might have provoked conflict and division within the
organization. However, the long-distance nature of the relationships
and the one-to-one conversations about the issue created no strife or
negative aftereffects among DSIN chapter leaders and national leaders.
The difference of opinion between me and Murdock-Vaughan did not
escalate into dissension at this time.

There were two different agendas exerting pressure on DSIN's
official position: (1) the need to stand up boldly on matters of fairness and justice and (2) respect for the needs of the approximately
200,000 women in this case, not simply the wishes of a few. As DSIN
evolved, we were responding to the needs of the women who contacted us and synthesizing what we heard them saying, continually
reframing our agenda around that discourse.

One reason I was receptive to this press conference plan from
Group B was that their lawyer/advisor spoke confidently about the
joint participation, at the press conference, of two nationally prominent public figures and some prominent Dalkon Shield lawyers. The
participation of these prominent figures would boost enormously what
I perceived as a very risky protest. We perceived the endeavor as risky
because so many people, including Dalkon Shield claimants, wanted

a settlement of any kind, under almost any terms. DSIN agreed to facilitate introductions between Group B and the DSAC women based in Vancouver and to invite the Canadian group to participate in the press conference also. The Canadian women were enthusiastic about joining this event. DSIN also offered to solicit Kathy Bonk's help with media coverage.

After a tentative agreement was reached on these matters, Group B's lawyer/advisor then lobbied to include, as a speaker, a woman we had never heard of before. According to him, this woman had started an organization for Dalkon Shield victims in California. It turned out that she was a lawyer, not a Dalkon Shield survivor, and that her group was defunct. I did not agree to have her as a speaker, on the grounds that our opposition to the plan was very risky and that including her at this juncture would greatly increase the risks. Group B's lawyer/advisor invited this woman to Washington despite my objections.

On the day before the press conference, all the groups gathered in Bonk's Washington offices to plan the final content of the press conference. She and members of her staff gave important and generous advice about how to structure and execute the event. She had already spent much time and many resources on the advance press for the event. She had persuaded many of her national media contacts to cover this press conference.

There were approximately 12 participants at the table during the planning, including members of the three Dalkon Shield groups, lawyers, and Bonk's staff. The assembled group was completely disorganized and fought long into the night over the choice of speakers and the content of the press conference. I came to the table with the expectation that each group would make its autonomous statement in opposition to the plan. This is how all DSIN-sponsored press conferences had been executed. I brought to this press conference a prepared statement that reflected the DSIN position, as mentioned previously, recommending modifications to the reorganization plan.

The other groups at this planning session lobbied for a united front of total opposition to the plan. I felt a deep conflict between my duty to all the DSIN chapter leaders and the dynamics of the current situation with these other groups. I felt under double duress because our actions now were important in determining how the cause would be perceived by a wider set of prominent people in the women's movement whom we saw as having the potential to be our greatest allies and helpers. In the end, I agreed to a unified *no* vote on the plan. I felt co-opted and I agonized over, even regretted, this course of action. I was insistent that, if lawyers were to speak at the event, they very clearly identify themselves as lawyers, and that they make their own statement apart from the women's groups.

The press conference was extremely successful, due to the skillful interventions and assistance of Bonk. The preparations, however, had been grueling. Murdock-Vaughan observed that we had all acted like a badly dysfunctional family. We fought with one another bitterly "off camera" but put on a convincing "front" during the press conference and individual interviews with the press. Bonk commented that she was disheartened by the strife and all the mistrust, but she remarked at how familiar it was to her from her many years in the feminist movement. Based on her long experience with antagonistic factions in the women's movement, she advised that the three groups find a way to form a permanent coalition. From her perspective, the problem of the male lawyers' involvement was not an insurmountable obstacle.

Bonk offered to continue to facilitate and mediate the ongoing work of this coalition, including offering to arrange a direct-mail campaign, with the *pro bono* assistance of fundraising professionals within her own network. This was another major gesture of sorely needed assistance. That mailing would have gone out to more than 20,000 Dalkon Shield claimants. She even drew up a skeleton outline for an immediate, nationwide media barnstorming blitz across the country that would urge Dalkon Shield claimants to reject the reorganization plan.

Murdock-Vaughan, Reeck, and I spent several days after the press conference agonizing over this advice. There were tense and strained discussions among the three of us. Murdock-Vaughan and Reeck wanted to join in a coalition.

> Surviving in the world of the white male power structure is not possible if we withdraw from the fight at this moment. If we do that, they win. Besides, this is the big chance we have wanted to learn from women who have really been powerful and successful. (Cinders Murdock-Vaughan)

Written notes that Murdock-Vaughan kept during this time indicate that I alternated, on a daily basis, between agreeing to and rejecting the coalition plan. There were several reasons for my objections to this coalition: (1) the continuing visceral distrust for the lawyer/advisor of Group B and suspicion of a possible "hidden agenda," (2) a fear of losing control of the grass-roots/survivors' campaign, which had been quite successful up to this point; and (3) an intense, and mostly irrational, fear of attack or death threats.

Murdock-Vaughan, Reeck, and I shared a perception that the women leaders of Group B were still not directing their organization more independently of their lawyer/advisor. I was also unable to let go of my anger that he had included someone new in the press conference despite my express objections. Considering those two points, I was convinced that he would attempt to dominate any coalition. A coalition might have had some promise of reaching and perhaps unifying a larger number of Dalkon Shield women, but in my judgment the composition of this particular coalition was too problematic. For Murdock-Vaughan and Reeck, it seemed manageable in the manner that Bonk assured.

> I wanted desperately to use that format for us to grow bigger and faster and have a greater impact, and I thought we would have to compromise somewhat for the greater good. In the long range, I thought that would be worthwhile. (Donna Reeck)

I was unwilling to compromise what I perceived to be DSIN's integrity for whatever expansion may have been possible. I would not cooperate with what I felt was a move to weaken the overall women's movement. For me, there were too many signs of male domination, with other, hidden agendas. As I stated in a memorandum to all potential coalition members on May 10, 1988:

> Our independent, claimant identity has been very successful for DSIN. [Mr. X], with his lawyer visibility in [Group B], and now in the other claimant organizations as a result of the press conference, will jeopardize the "greater good" and that is a risk DSIN is not willing to take.

I invoked the name of the organization to discuss the risk, even though there was clearly no consensus within DSIN. In the end, for me, this particular configuration for a permanent coalition was unworkable. I was uncompromising. Murdock-Vaughan and Reeck did not challenge my decision or demand the outcome that they supported. This event did lead to organizational problems, which are discussed under "DSIN Power Structure" in Chapter 5. It is ironic that, in our desperate quest to establish relationships with others, a relationship issue caused the greatest strain for DSIN leadership.

I was not familiar with the literature on social movements at the time of these events, but later, after reading Blumberg and West's (1989) conclusion about women who participate in social movements, I felt validated about my decision on the coalition. In other cases of women's social protest that they studied, women's roles got lost when success increased. "Women often initiate protest on the local level. As the organizations grow and develop power, men assume or are even encouraged to assume formal leadership positions" (p. 10).

In the final analysis, that coalition did not accomplish the agenda originally outlined during the press conference of May 1988. Group B did continue to collaborate with DSAC, the Canadian group, but, according to correspondence sent by DSAC leaders to DSIN, DSAC found the subsequent relationships frustrating and not egalitarian (E. Cumley, personal communication, October 24, 1988).

DSIN used the terms *ally* and *friend* to refer to other organizations. The outside world perceives that the cooperating groups of a coalition have an equal status and that a coalition shifts, or redefines, the identities of all groups that belong to it. A coalition may even dilute the distinct identities of each member group. This factor contributed to my refusal to be a member of this particular coalition.

It had been extremely important for DSIN to cultivate allies and friends who supported and endorsed DSIN actions and with whom we could have a relationship of reciprocity and equality. Group B began its life with ambitious organizational goals beyond those involving the Dalkon Shield. The action agenda of DSIN evolved incrementally, from absorbing and synthesizing the shared experience of persons involved with the group, working more from the "gut" than from ideology or doctrine. The content and rhetoric of DSIN activism emerged from the collective voices of Dalkon Shield survivors. In fact, I began my activism in DSIN—as did others—with a notion that destroying the wealth of the Robins Company through some means, perhaps a boycott, would shift the emphasis of this case from money to the violation of human rights. I modified my personal desires and goals as I met scores of other survivors and got deeply involved in the complexity of the issues.

At the beginning of DSIN activism, the public posture of the group was largely reactive; that is, it countered or criticized Robins. In due time, DSIN began to develop a proactive agenda, making its own demands for a fair and just outcome. DSIN leaders felt adamantly that women who were survivors of this reproductive disaster should have their own concerns and views of justice included in the public forum, in their own voices. DSIN leaders also felt that although lawyers can and do play important roles in social movements, for which they should be embraced, their presence and influence in a grass-roots organization should be restricted or limited to an advisory, not a leadership, capacity and their identities as lawyers should be disclosed.

THE COURT

Litigation surrounding this case was more than a decade old by the time women survivors began advocating for themselves. When they first became active in the organization, very few DSIN members had any knowledge of the court system, rules, or protocol, much less the nuances and implicit subtleties of the legal subculture. We learned legal technicalities through a relentless pursuit of information. We were self-taught. After two years of involvement, some DSIN leaders were more knowledgeable about bankruptcy law than some personal-injury lawyers, several of whom, who had no previous experience in this type of litigation, contacted us for information.

The first DSIN protest actions were scheduled outside the courtroom, on the courthouse steps. Later, DSIN members began to attend pivotal court hearings and eventually learned how to insert at least some claimants' concerns directly into the official court record. DSIN insinuated itself into a process that did not ask for its contributions.

> I was so overwhelmed that there was so little representation of women in the courtroom. I could count them on one hand. I was appalled that men were controlling us again. I felt slightly powerless, and if I felt powerless, it's because somewhere I handed that power over to someone else. (Donna Reeck)

As detailed in Chapter 3, many obstacles stood in the way of women's direct participation in the Robins bankruptcy litigation. From the official standpoint, Dalkon Shield claimants were represented by a duly authorized Claimants' Committee, a standard procedure for all stakeholder groups in Chapter 11 proceedings.[6] In general, legal language was an imposing barrier. It is a professional jargon that is almost impenetrable to cultural outsiders. Additionally, the court did not acknowledge the early proposal for an information and support service (discussed in Chapter 3), public access to the claimant mailing list was first denied and then made prohibitively expensive, and litigants were legally prohibited from meeting directly with the presiding judge.

The bankruptcy court also made communication in the opposite direction difficult, for example, by prohibiting the Claimants' Committee from sending an informational letter on the status of the case to all claimants (Sobol, 1991). Women with strong determination, fairly good literacy skills, and persistence eventually found out who their Dalkon Shield advocates were by reading the national newspapers. Many women attempted to establish communication with the Claimants' Committee, as I did. There were three women claimants on the official five-member Claimants' Committee: Two were bankruptcy lawyers and the third was a college professor.[7] The Claimants' Committee at this time was represented in the courtroom and the negotiations by the law firm of Cadwalader, Wickersham, and Taft.

Once familiar with the legal language and in possession of some rudimentary working knowledge of the court's rituals, DSIN began to submit its own documents to the court, as lawyers were doing. DSIN leaders got to know countless plaintiffs' lawyers who were involved in the litigation. Conversations with scores of those lawyers were distilled into strategies for getting into the official record. At the time DSIN began entering the courtroom, very few Dalkon Shield women attended the hearings; however, more women began to attend the hearings during the course of DSIN activism. The DSIN newsletter advertised the hearing dates and encouraged members to attend.

Women who were part of DSIN began taking voluminous notes on the content of the hearings.[8] This improved our ability to speak to the issues. DSIN shifted its initial strategy of holding press conferences during the hearings and began holding press conferences *after* attending the hearings. This allowed us to formulate an informed commentary on and reaction to the latest developments as they happened. On every trip to Richmond, DSIN leaders tried to meet with as many Richmond parties as possible who were formally involved in the case, always asking for clarification and volunteering DSIN member opinions on the latest developments. DSIN leaders always pressed for details on the ways in which the Dalkon Shield claimants were being treated during the negotiations. The goal of all this activity was to demonstrate indirectly to Judge Merhige, through the people he did interact with formally, that the entire case was of serious and vital interest to Dalkon Shield women.

The group estimation on the total value of all the claims was a critical piece of information women needed to determine how their individual claims would eventually be assessed by the Trust. Each of the seven stakeholder groups presented its own estimation at this three-day hearing. Robins offered the lowest estimate range ($698 million to $1.2 billion) and the Dalkon Shield Claimants Committee offered the highest estimate range ($4 billion to $7 billion). At the end of the hearing on this issue, Judge Merhige issued findings in support of the $2.475 billion estimate for the aggregate claims (Sobol, 1991, p. 230) and stated unequivocally that there would be enough money to pay all valid claims. He did not issue written findings, making it impossible for us to determine his method for reaching that conclusion. We had determined, by listening closely to the courtroom testimony, that pertinent information about the individual value of the claims could be extracted from the testimony, so we requested (and received) the relevant documents from Robins's lawyers.

In an effort to demonstrate an increasingly serious involvement by some Dalkon Shield claimants in the legal process, DSIN held a Richmond conference for all DSIN leaders in February 1988 and formally invited Judge Merhige to address the group. (See Chapter 3.) Prior to the event, Merhige declined in writing to appear, but he arranged for us to tour the Dalkon Shield claims resolution facility. In the end, he made a surprise appearance and talked to the group during the tour. We saw this unexpected meeting with Judge Merhige as a symbolic acknowledgment of DSIN women and their seriousness of purpose. Paul Barrett, the *Wall Street Journal* reporter who was writing most of the stories on the case at the time, had asked to attend the DSIN conference, accompanied us throughout the weekend's activities, and interviewed a large number of DSIN chapter leaders. Barrett eventually wrote a feature article on the case and the events of that conference (Barrett, 1988).

The only other direct interactions between Judge Merhige and DSIN leaders took place during two different court hearings, when DSIN objections were presented orally during the March 1988 hearing and were scheduled to be presented in July 1988 at the confirmation hearing. However, Judge Merhige refused to allow me to present DSIN objections at the July 18 plan confirmation hearing. When I challenged him and refused to sit down, he angrily ordered the federal marshals to remove me from the courtroom. (See Chapter 3 for a full account.)

The vote gave a resounding, landslide approval of the reorganization plan. The DSIN objection was clearly a tiny minority opinion, but Merhige denied its entry into the official court record. Perhaps he felt that objections from any claimants blemished an otherwise superbly orchestrated strategy to have this plan go down in history as one that the claimants themselves, by their 94% approval vote, agreed was the best solution to this precedent-setting case of mass tort litigation.

Judge Merhige's handling of the Dalkon Shield case has been criticized as unethical and biased by several observers and lawyers close to this litigation. The records and documentation of this massive litigation now contain evidence that Judge Merhige was having unofficial *ex parte* meetings with Robins officials and many other parties to the case (Bragg, 1986; Mintz, 1986a; Sobol, 1991). A number of plaintiffs' lawyers have charged that he had been biased and vengeful during the proceedings and that he violated legal ethics by meeting with one side (of lawyers) in the absence of representatives from all sides (Labaton, 1988b; Sobol, 1991).

Merhige enforced his authority over this case in a classic patriarchal manner. Judge Merhige has even been dubbed the *father* of the settlement plan by one of the (male) Dalkon Shield trustees (Labaton, 1988a). Judge Merhige ran his courtroom with strict rules, including prohibitions against gum chewing and reading magazines. On several occasions, Dalkon Shield women were told to spit out gum or leave the courtroom. Sobol confirms the feeling of that rigid domination that women experienced and observed inside the courtroom. "Merhige takes his role as the presiding officer quite seriously, and he is a stickler for enforcing courtroom decorum and deference to his authority" (Sobol, 1991, p. 194). At the hearings that drew large numbers of lawyers and women, entry into the courtroom was restricted.

> In the courtroom, it was kind of humiliating, the way we had to take turns [to get a seat inside], wait for seats, and we ended up sitting in the jury box. We were claimants and that was humiliating, that they made no provisions for us to take part or to be able to at least hear what was going on. (Jan Thompson)

Judge Merhige routinely exhibited anger and hostility during the hearings, directing caustic, biting verbal attacks at Dalkon Shield claimants' attorneys. In our perception, he ridiculed Dalkon Shield claimant advocates repeatedly. Excerpts from court transcripts and anecdotes in Richard Sobol's (1991) book also confirm this hostility. DSIN members who attended hearings never observed his biting sarcasm directed at Robins's counsel or witnesses. In the episode already mentioned when he had me removed from the courtroom, I perceived his angry demeanor as harshly paternalistic, as if he were meting out punishment for a child's bad behavior. This treatment enraged me. When he fired Ann Samani, the only claimant trustee of the Trust, he cited her *open defiance* of the court's authority (Sobol, 1991).[9]

THE LAWYERS

Trial lawyers mediate the legal system for victims.[10] In the course of three years, DSIN leaders and representatives would develop some degree of relations or interaction with about 50 lawyers actively involved in the litigation. (According to Mike Sheppard, there are more than 8,000 lawyers representing women's claims before the claimants' Trust.) Many of those lawyers participated intensely and enduringly in this case, including years of litigation before the bankruptcy proceeding began. A handful of lawyers gave generously of their time, teaching us legal principles and subtle intricacies of the case, sending us legal documents that we requested, and so forth. Some even subscribed to our newsletter. We received no more than 25 small donations (in amounts ranging from $15 to $100) from lawyers throughout these three years.

In the experience of DSIN leaders, lawyers were divided into two groups: "white hats" and those who were not. DSIN leaders used a single criterion to define a lawyer as a *white hat*: that the lawyer demonstrate a primary interest in the issues of justice and basic fairness involved in this case, not a simple focus on compensation. DSIN leaders and members assessed lawyers, based on first impressions, using this guideline. Lawyers who addressed the larger issues of justice (in the courtroom, in written literature, or during conversations with us) were assessed as, in general, more trustworthy. Some lawyers were indeed actively concerned with those larger issues of justice that concerned us greatly. Bob Manchester had worked hard to get a worldwide recall of the Dalkon Shield (see Chapter 2). Douglas Bragg and Bradley Post sought to recuse Judge Merhige from the case, due to what they considered to be biased and unethical conduct on his part (as discussed previously). They also confronted other lawyers about the ethically controversial "wholesaling" and brokering of cases. Other lawyers filed motions to have the litigation moved out of Richmond, Robins's hometown.

DSIN leaders modified their opinions and positions on lawyers as a result of interacting with them directly throughout these three years and hearing women's reports of various negative experiences. At the beginning of our involvement, we did not perceive it a major problem that lawyers handling these cases would be financially compensated. However, after DSIN leaders had met scores of the lawyers involved in this case, we became increasingly uncomfortable and even angry with those we thought to be motivated solely by their own aggrandizement. We saw in their behavior the same greed that had motivated Robins and precipitated this senseless health disaster by abusing women. The potential for revictimization is substantial; perhaps some women will be victimized *again* at any cost.

The evidence we accumulated to make assessments about lawyers comes from the experiences reported to us from women who contacted DSIN. Some examples cited below demonstrate the range of conduct we encountered—the negative value systems, which we abhorred and believed posed a threat of further victimization, as well as the positive professionalism that we respected.

1. Many women report being told by some of the prominent Dalkon Shield lawyers that their cases were not "good enough," not worthy of that lawyer's time. Although it is true that some women do not have "good" cases (i.e., some women do not have the medical documentation necessary to support their claims), it is the manner in which the women have been treated that is disturbing. It felt a lot like degradation and devaluation of their human dignity. Women who reported these events were enraged by the treatment they had received.

2. The fact that one lawyer engaged in behavior toward DSIN leaders that left us feeling intimidated set an early tone for distrust and skepticism toward all lawyers. (See the previous section in this chapter entitled "Conflicts and Confrontations.") This feeling was modified as we learned who the "white hats" were.

3. When public access to the mailing list of all claimants finally became available for the outrageously high price of $82,877 (Sobol, 1991), lawyers purchased regional sections of the list and solicited clients, a practice considered ethically controversial within the law profession. Some lawyers even sold sections of the lists they purchased to other lawyers, and women reported receiving two or three different solicitation letters (Gladwell, 1989). One newspaper story portrays the fierce competition among lawyers for clients. One attorney accused another attorney of conducting an improper direct-mail campaign.

> Thornton, who represents claimants in the United States, Canada, and Europe, said Medical Legal Consultants joined with law firms and law-

yers in other cities last year in the largest mass mailing ever in the United States to solicit clients in a legal action. Those firms and lawyers, who lent their names to provide local connections, agreed to finance the mailing for part of the eventual fees even though they may have had no direct role in the case. (Miletich, 1989, p. A7)

The other attorney denied the allegations. Another article describes how Thornton traveled around the country to more than 25 U.S. cities and parts of Canada, Puerto Rico, and Ireland over a 1½-year period, "holding press conferences and seminars to provide legal help to victims without lawyers" (Gladwell, 1989, p. H8). Not surprisingly, this strategy also resulted in hundreds, if not thousands, of clients for Thornton.

   Yet, in spite of all the lawyers' advertising and marketing efforts, approximately 60% of the 113,000 "active" claimants did not have legal representation as of January 1990, according to Julie Freeman, manager of claimant relations at the Trust. It is hard to know why the vast majority did not hire lawyers, but our experience led us to posit several possible reasons: (a) The court told women, in the very first mail they sent to claimants, that they did not have to hire a lawyer[11]—women simply took that advice at face value; (b) the general public has become increasingly skeptical about and distrustful of the legal profession, particularly personal-injury lawyers; and (c) the women simply trusted the court officials to do the right thing in paying on their claims.

4. Women reported that after the bankruptcy proceeding moved toward the establishment of a capped trust fund (a finite amount of money set aside to compensate all Dalkon Shield claimants), some lawyers increased their contingency fees from the standard 33% to as much as 50% or 60%. On the other hand, other lawyers promised that they would reduce their fees for representing claims in the "lower" ranges of value. The latter was a double-edged sword, however. There are honorable, respectable lawyers reducing their fees for the lower claims values; however, there were also lawyers whose marketing plan was to accumulate a large number of less serious claims. This is what we came to call "the H&R Block approach." The phenomenon has been described slightly differently by Sobol (1991):

   Other lawyers—generally those who had advertised—had hundreds of clients. . . . They were in favor of an alternative dispute resolution mechanism that would provide a rapid and relatively expeditious means of disposing of cases, even if the dispositions were not of the highest possible value. These two schools of thought came to be known as the "retailers" and the "wholesalers." (p. 73)

An article in the *Washington Post*, featuring a lawyer named Andrew Zieve, highlights this phenomenon.

Already, Zieve represents 1,000 Shield victims, and, as a result of an aggressive marketing campaign, he has another dozen calling every day. Some estimate the average award to each victim at between $25,000 and $75,000, which means that Zieve's share of the Dalkon trust fund will be—conservatively—$8 million. If he's lucky, it's triple that. (Gladwell, 1989, p. H8)

Another attorney has spoken often of the enormous personal debt he has assumed to prepare for his more than 1,500 cases: "[In the beginning], we were all basically idealistic, and we felt that Robins did some terrible things. But now it is a business. . . . We've been forced to become more entrepreneurial" (Gladwell, 1989, p. H8).

For many DSIN members, the overall effect of absorbing this "business" made us feel that Dalkon Shield women were considered little more than bricks paving the road to the pot of gold at the rainbow's end. It left many of us with a sick and dehumanized feeling. When we made discouraging discoveries such as this, our optimism at low ebb, we often shared a dark vision of scores of people conjuring up ways to make a buck on Dalkon Shield misery.

5. Some lawyers did not keep their clients informed about the bankruptcy proceedings. Women also report that their lawyers never forwarded them any mail from Richmond, not even a copy of the reorganization plan that was mailed to all claimants, and many women did not even know that they had the right to vote on the reorganization plan. They were not consulted about how they wanted their attorneys to cast their votes. On the other hand, other attorneys did send newsletters, full of quality information, and these lawyers even encouraged women to instruct them on how to cast their vote on the plan for them.

Kidder and Fine (1986) provide an apt context for describing the strained relations between Dalkon Shield activists and some of these lawyers. The authors distinguish between *conflict-of-interest* and *missed-opportunities* perspectives for framing analyses of social injustice. In the first type, a *group* analyzes injustice structurally and defines it as a collective problem. Actors identify the opposition and then engage in a fight for outcomes that they will control rather than ask for help that is controlled by authorities. Grass-roots political groups, such as DSIN, focus on the conflict-of-interests perspective and use collective action to find solutions.

From the perspective of missed opportunities, problems are perceived to be individual and anomalous, which means that the solutions are defined, controlled, and delivered by trained professionals (the experts) who have the power and legitimate authority to help the deserving individuals (the clients). This model is also based on meritocracy, with individual outcomes deriving from personal efforts. In general, Western culture highly prizes these values.

The experts (in this case, lawyers) can promote victim-blaming ideologies that maintain inequitable power structures and convince dissenters that they are angry, crazy, fragile, or overly sensitive (Kidder & Fine, 1986). They may even collude in trivializing injuries. One prominent Dalkon Shield lawyer enraged DSIN leaders with his public assessment of the damages: "They tell you they've gone through hell for years, but often it's pain and bleeding and nothing more" (Barrett, 1988, p. 29). "Pain and bleeding" is the term for an explicit category of legal damages involving the lowest level of monetary award. This lawyer undoubtedly was thinking about this connotation of the term when he made these remarks. Countless Dalkon Shield users, however, were enraged by this statement, which seemed to trivialize the very real pain and bleeding they had suffered for more than a decade.

These structural arrangements sustain power differentials between victims and the formal institutions of power. As clients in the missed-opportunities model, victims remain isolated from one another and the victimization is kept private. Lawyers are their agents, mediating a frightening and complex system for them. Some of these lawyers keep victims passive, dependent, and uninformed.[12] They are also the brokers for the court authorities in exercising control over the "victims." The use of the term *victim* became increasingly offensive to us because of its connotations of helplessness, powerlessness, and pity. We insisted on referring to ourselves as "survivors" and felt that what we were doing for ourselves had transformed the sense of personal trauma.

For lawyers who subscribed to the missed-opportunities model, the collective energies and actions of DSIN were a threat. Some women who called the DSIN hotline reported that their lawyers instructed them not to get in touch with DSIN. Such lawyers are part of the patriarchal hegemony that perpetuates inequities like those that characterize the Dalkon Shield case. During the first year of activism, DSIN leaders felt that they had been intimidated by one of these personal-injury lawyers. (See the section earlier in this chapter entitled "Conflicts and Confrontations.") This same lawyer sent us a letter after our public opposition to the reorganization plan, mentioning the prospect of "penalties" against us, which again made us feel as if we were being intimidated.

DSIN relations with a large number of lawyers in this case did allow us to draw the conclusion that there are many good lawyers fighting hard on this issue who actually are responsible for bringing this case as much into the public domain as possible. We became disenchanted and conflicted, however, by the emphasis on business and personal wealth, topics that were discussed by some of these lawyers in such a matter-of-fact manner. More lawyers need to work to change the legal system so that comparable gross social injustices involving medical drugs and devices do not continue to occur. Unfortunately, the incidence of corporate misconduct and dangerous products seems to be increasing. The program booklet from the 1992 American Trial Lawyers Association annual conference indicates a current array of more than 70 different litigation specialties—13 of which involve pharmaceutical products.

The DSIN response to the dilemmas and controversies surrounding lawyers evolved and changed over time, as we heard from women who had had varying degrees of positive and negative experiences with individual lawyers. At first, we developed a list of the six to eight lawyers with whom we had had our earliest, most congenial interactions. Feedback from women about them, however, was mixed; some of them had bad experiences, and this made us feel that our own credibility was in jeopardy for recommending some of these lawyers.

As a result of indications that women might be treated poorly or even abused, we consulted other public interest organizations about how to proceed. We obtained materials from an organization called HALT—An Organization of Americans for Legal Reform. This group was attempting to educate the public about how to deal with lawyers. They had published a handbook titled "Using a Lawyer . . . and What to Do If Things Go Wrong." As a result of our consultations, we developed a set of guidelines that advised women on how to evaluate and negotiate with a lawyer regarding the Dalkon Shield issue. We told them to negotiate for a reduced fee, since their claims were not going to be handled in the standard manner. Rather than become embroiled in either lawyer praising or lawyer bashing, DSIN opted to provide information that encouraged women to empower themselves to resolve their needs regarding legal representation.

Also, early on, we felt that the circumstance was so complex that women needed lawyers to protect their claims. The lack of access to information cited above and detailed in Sobol's (1991) book caused many people, including us, to worry that women might get knocked out of the process completely by inadvertently giving the wrong information on the early questionnaires from the court. For example, questions about the statute of limitations are particularly puzzling to people who are not well schooled in the legal requirements. Some women were determined not to hire lawyers and did substantial legal homework on how to process their own claims. They were the exception. Most women simply placed their trust in the court and the Trust to protect them. As mentioned above, more than half the claimants did not acquire legal representation.[13]

At first DSIN did not take a position on lawyers' fees. When we began to hear anecdotes of fees exceeding the standard 33% contingency fee, we grappled with an appropriate response to this dilemma. One alternative to private representation that Jan Thompson (DSIN–Colorado) explored with Nancy Davis, formerly a claimant member of the Claimants' Committee, and Nadine Taub, of the Rutgers Women's Rights Litigation Clinic, was the development of legal clinics, to be operated out of university law schools with staff trained to assist women in filing the required paperwork to submit their claims, for a modest fee, or for free, if grant monies could be secured. Women with large claims would be advised to seek an attorney.

Another idea was to file a motion with the court recommending a limit, or "cap," on legal fees. Throughout the bankruptcy proceedings, Judge Merhige made continuous references to high legal fees, and rumors buzzed that he would be receptive to such a motion. This had the potential to become the most explosive and contentious issue in the entire bankruptcy litigation. I feel quite sure that if a cap on lawyers' fees had been codified as part of the Trust's protocols, lawyers would have rallied to defeat the reorganization plan. The contingency fee system provides average people a fundamental access to the civil justice system, a privilege not found in many other countries, and it is central to the survival of personal-injury lawyers.

Although we supported the idea of regulating fees in spirit, based on the instances of abuse that women were reporting to us and from what we knew about certain lawyers' schemes to attract clients, DSIN decided not to tackle this issue. We did not have adequate resources or enough legal advocates of our own to cope with what would have been monstrous repercussions from lawyers. We were also ambivalent about the whole issue, because we did not trust the court system to do the right thing. We did not consider challenging this issue as a viable option for our group.

In sum, the relationship between lawyers and grass-roots activists is a complex one. Lawyers need to identify themselves separately from the grass-roots, activist organizations, especially when public activities are being coordinated among groups. They should not create self-serving nonprofit organizations, which most certainly are not grass-roots-inspired. The consequences of lawyers remaining submerged (manipulating behind the scenes) within a social movement are the contamination and delegitimizing of the victims' voices and issues, as well as a continuing societal hostility toward lawyers as a group.

Societal sentiment is increasingly hostile toward personal-injury lawyers, a hostility that was exacerbated by the Reagan and Bush administrations' claims of a so-called litigation crisis. Lawyers were blamed for stifling innovations and new product development (including contraceptives), leaving the United States ill equipped to compete adequately in the global marketplace (McQueen, 1989; Sugarman, 1990). Yet data from credible and well-established organizations within the business world itself do not confirm the existence of runaway litigation (Conference Board, Inc., 1987; Schmitt, 1989).

Lawyers have made valuable and necessary contributions to social movements. The Dalkon Shield case is considered to be one of the most complex personal-injury, or "mass tort," cases ever to enter the legal system. Myriad issues emanate from the precedents set in this litigation, including the power and authority of the errant corporations to determine the final solutions, the lack of criminal punishment for the corporate perpetrators of the crime, the threat to compensation rights for victims of future mass torts, and the exoneration of co-conspirators (such as the insurance industry), to name a few. Ideally, activists and lawyers should find some way to collaborate on some of these issues.

THE MEDICAL WORLD

Physicians and the health care system, in general, have not supported the resolution of this social injustice to women; in fact, they are entirely absent, publicly, as advocates for women. In the 1970s, a handful of concerned doctors did bring the problems with this medical device to the attention of Congress, which resulted in the congressional hearings on IUDs (Committee on Government Operations, 1973). These doctors lobbied to have the Shield removed from the marketplace. But since that time almost 20 years ago, there have been only a handful of medical advocates for Dalkon Shield women in the public forum. Physicians were hired as consultants to analyze and assess the value of the claims during the formal court proceedings, but physicians' formal professional organizations are notably absent from and silent on public support for the victims of this tragedy.

DSIN attempted to establish relationships with medical and health professionals. Through other Dalkon Shield women, DSIN leaders did make some personal contacts with a total of four or five physicians who were willing to attend DSIN meetings, write columns in the DSIN newsletter, and go on television to talk about the medical problems from which Dalkon Shield women suffered. Only infertility specialists supported us in any demonstrable way. They were in great demand by women who, in desperation to become pregnant, resorted to the then-new high-tech infertility treatments, such as *in vitro* fertilization. To my knowledge, doctors did not publicly address the political issue and the social injustice. I believe that the hysteria surrounding liability accounts for physicians' lack of public or political involvement on behalf of women damaged by the Shield.

Some women reported that their doctors would not even cooperate with their attempts to gather their medical records. Several factors compounded this situation. First, the original injuries had happened so long ago that records were now missing, incomplete, or purged. Doctors in many states are required to keep records for only a limited number of years, and in many states, that limit is seven years. Second, a close scrutiny of records might have uncovered medical malpractice in connection with the aftermath of this defective medical device. For example, Gloria Manago (DSIN–North Carolina) eventually suffered six miscarriages, with increasing severity of hemorrhage and life-threatening effects each time. The details of her story indicate serious mismanagement of her problems.

An analysis of the range of problems associated with acquiring medical documentation would be a valuable contribution to the literature on the magnitude of medical abuse of women. The dilemmas faced by Dalkon Shield users, who tried to reconstruct their medical histories 10, 15, and even 20 years later, make a compelling case for a complete overhaul of the way medical records are treated. People should amass their own personal medical histories *at the time* they receive any form of medical attention, and they should keep a complete file of all their medical records in their own safekeeping. I also believe people should keep records of every pharmaceutical medication they ever consumed. Reconstructing medical histories many years after treatment is virtually impossible. The current system clearly benefits doctors over patients. In many instances, our health care system deliberately refuses people the right to their medical records. The lack of medical records was the chief reason so many Dalkon Shield claims were disqualified by the court and the Trust.

In sum, the glaring lack of medical advocates, coupled with the posture of those who would deny the damage, only reconfirms and intensifies the early rage that many Dalkon Shield women developed when they discovered their original betrayal by the medical and health care system.

SUMMARY

DSIN began its life seeking help from what were perceived to be sophisticated, successful organizations concerned with a variety of related themes: reproductive rights, feminism, consumer affairs, other victims, and public interest legal groups. Feminist groups were particularly sought out because of their perceived role-model status in waging a fight against abusive institutions of power. In retrospect, there was not much acceptance and mutuality forthcoming to Dalkon Shield activists from the organized feminist movement. The most enduring and tension-free relationships have evolved with other victims' and human rights organizations.

With regard to all the formal and court-authorized parties to this case, DSIN leaders were unwelcome in the formal process. That did not stop the leaders from insinuating themselves into the official business. Some DSIN activity was intended to reach the judge indirectly through these other parties. Most of the communications with other official parties went one-way, from DSIN to the receiving end.

DSIN was *about* creating a community and a set of social relations to challenge the official worldview of elites. Before this, Dalkon Shield women were submerged in a culture of silence, with lawyers their only intermediaries with the formal institutions of power.

5 Analysis of the Movement

This chapter analyzes the movement's philosophical basis, early strategies, leadership profiles and development, accomplishments, successes, and limitations. The analysis of the group's embryonic phase is enhanced by interviews that were conducted with several DSIN leaders. Additionally, four of the women interviewed agreed to read and react to early drafts of the analysis, and their responses affirmed my analysis.

Ruzek (1978) charges that sociologists have largely ignored the role of women's social movements in social change due to the male dominance of social science. Social reform movements involving large numbers of women are not studied as seriously as political revolutions, which are usually organized and controlled by men. Ruzek charges that social science has been sexist in ignoring the role of women in these matters.

Social movements are political. The notion that social protest is something different from electoral politics is false. I concur with Ackelsberg (1988), who implores social science to change its conceptual framework for labeling and describing the political actions of women's groups such as the one described in this book. Scholars should enhance the status and prestige of women's organizations as dynamic, contemporary political organizations. Political life is not limited to electoral politics.

DSIN began as a relatively solitary quest for information. What evolved was the public and political construction of a community that had been submerged for almost 20 years. The goals of DSIN were to interrupt the culture of silence, to introduce the issues of this population of former Dalkon Shield users into the public discourse, and to wage a fight for justice as construed by the Dalkon Shield survivors themselves. The protest agenda and actions of DSIN women came to challenge the accountability of the legal system in living up to its own ideals.

The actions of these Dalkon Shield survivors were no less political in intent and consequences than the behavior of the lawyers, the corporate and insurance company executives, and the judge sitting on this case. DSIN attempted to become an advocate for the needs of the largest number of victims, including but not limited to economically disadvantaged women, chronically ill women, women who were prematurely disqualified from the Trust, and women of other nations. Women's letters to DSIN and telephone contacts were absorbed and synthesized, and then incorporated into the public agenda and discourse of DSIN leaders.

The terms *power* and *politics* have expanded meanings in the discourse on social injustice and mobilization efforts to ameliorate cases involving human rights. As defined by Hartsock (1979) and Miller (1986), power involves not only domination of others but also the capacity to implement and the energy to accomplish a goal. Power is not only something groups *have*, it is also a social relationship between groups that determines access to, use of, and control over the basic material and ideological resources in society (Bookman & Morgen, 1988).

This expanded definition of power encompasses the experience of the women who were part of the Dalkon Shield protest movement. From the moment of the group's creation, the women of DSIN were engaged in politics. This group began to emerge when people defined their condition as an intolerable injustice rather than as a misfortune warranting charitable consideration (Ruzek, 1978). A perception of injustice as a collective problem enables people to fight for outcomes they will control rather than ask for help that is controlled by authorities (Kidder & Fine, 1986).

DSIN was *about* creating a community and a set of social relations to challenge the official worldview that justice was being done to this population. Dalkon Shield injuries affected a large population of women, and public recognition of the magnitude of this health disaster could facilitate one of DSIN's long-term goals, that of lobbying other corporations and governmental agencies to work harder to prevent future health tragedies.

DSIN relied heavily, in its embryonic stage, on what can be called *relational* politics. The primary political strategy adopted by DSIN was the careful development and maintenance of particular sets of social relationships, both internally and externally. DSIN was deliberate about whom it identified with and whom it separated itself from in order to be representative, to the best of its ability, of the total community of Dalkon Shield victims. DSIN leaders began to develop a political action agenda by cultivating allies in other, more experienced public interest organizations. Through that process, DSIN leaders gained relevant skills and knowledge.

CONTEXTUAL PARAMETERS

As in any social movement, there were particular circumstances that affected both the emergence and shape of this Dalkon Shield protest movement. First, the A. H. Robins bankruptcy litigation in the mid-1980s presented a focal set of concrete events that set the stage for creating public awareness of the injured parties and the medical violence they had experienced. Except for congressional hearings in the late 1970s, which generated a modest amount of publicity, there had not been a significant opportunity to develop widespread awareness of this case until the bankruptcy proceedings. Once DSIN activists achieved wider attention to their interests, a sense of urgency and immediacy shaped the nature of the movement; that is, they developed strategies to "seize the moment" in pressing for their notions of justice by responding to the latest developments in the courtroom. DSIN came to fill a niche among the complex set of players in the political milieu in Richmond. We were the collective representation of the majority of Dalkon Shield women, and we were not representing any special interests. Prior to the emergence of DSIN, lawyers were the only agents for Dalkon Shield women with the elites who control the formal institutions of power.

Secondly, women injured by the Dalkon Shield were widely dispersed around the United States and the rest of the globe. These women were mostly unaware of the circumstances that had caused their individual problems until the bankruptcy proceedings began in 1985, requiring the Robins Company to mount a major publicity campaign. In this case, the sexual nature of the injuries and their sequelae presented a significant additional barrier for women to break through in order to seek information or to become public advocates for their own rights.

It has been noted by other observers of social movements that an organized clientele with a collective awareness of its constitutency can present a serious threat to authority (Ruzek, 1978). Professionals can then be observed and evaluated by clients who share some common values or expectations. Power elites fear public "naming" of their misbehavior and find critical conversation about social and economic arrangements a very dangerous situation (Fine, 1987). "Collectivities, especially articulate groups with access to the press, potentially wield power in democratic societies" (Ruzek, 1978, p. 180).

Dalkon Shield women and some of their advocates experienced substantial resistance from the power elites with regard to management of information and access to communication with the vast majority of other survivors. DSIN broke that barrier and was creative and persistent in using alternative strategies, particularly with the press, in order to overcome this obstacle.

Acknowledging the Rage at Betrayal

Most of the women who became part of this social movement were political amateurs; their activism did not emerge from any political philosophy or previous political experience. Their energies for this work emanated from rage about their loss of fertility and the violation of their bodies by a corporation that knowingly promoted a defective contraceptive. After absorbing and integrating this new information about the cause of their injuries, many of these women wanted to take action against the responsible corporate executives. The anger became a vehicle to empowerment. The most common theme among women who became DSIN leaders was deep bitterness and cynicism about a medical and legal system that tolerates and allows these kinds of senselesss tragedies.

> This bankruptcy thing has just been a big cover up. We have become the sacrificial lamb. If they give us justice, it would set precedents for other companies, and they don't want to do it because people are afraid of their money, their stocks. Start thinking about who gets hurt. That's the sad part. I was sold out for a dollar. (Joanne Ackerman)

> We should have milked them dry. Why should we care? They didn't care about our lives. They should have really gone bankrupt. They should have gone down the tubes. We should have been able to attach all their properties, their houses, their cars and everything else they own. It's been a rotten game of real bad politics. (Sherry Fletcher)

PHILOSOPHICAL FOUNDATIONS

Early on, DSIN members amassed the tales of horror and injustice from direct contact with hundreds of victims. The experiences expressed in those hundreds of letters and thousands of telephone contacts were synthesized into what would become the group's action agenda. DSIN hoped to make it possible for the multitude of women to come forward, to claim recognition in the public domain. DSIN leaders were quite successful in gaining legitimacy by articulating, in a general way, the needs and demands of this large population.

The philosophical foundations of this movement arose from three sources: (1) grief over the loss of fertility—the one high social status assigned to women in this society; (2) rage for the callous and willful violation of bodily intergrity; and (3) the aftereffects of being victimized and treated in a patronizing and subhuman fashion by various official institutions of power.

The Dalkon Shield injustice involved a violation of sacred reproductive rights. Without their consent, many Dalkon Shield users were robbed of the ability to bear children. Women's ability to reproduce—that is, their fertility status—is widely valued in society, including by the elites who control the formal institutions of power. "The core of being a woman is our reproductive rights. It should be the single most important thing to protect—the right to recreate life, and nurture it and watch it grow" (Donna Reeck).

Maternalism is one theme that emerges repeatedly to explain women's participation in all kinds of social protest (Blumberg & West, 1989).[1] Women's reasoning about social protest includes the feeling of a special mission regarding issues impacting their families' welfare (Blumberg & West, 1989). Some DSIN members speak of substituting this political activism for their mothering, or even their nurturing, needs:

> I needed to figure out a way to go on without having another baby. I saw this [DSIN] as being sort of creative and helpful and nurturing, like having a baby, and it made me feel good knowing that I was doing something important. (Jan Thompson)

However, maternalism is not a sufficient explanation. Another major motivation for women's activism is rage. In the Dalkon Shield case, the anger emanated from their egregious abuse by a medical system that subordinated women's welfare to the profit motive. Women wanted to seek revenge on A. H. Robins for this medical violence. They wanted to strike back and hurt the men and the company that had destroyed their bodies and obliterated their chances of motherhood.

Violent revenge fantasies directed at Dr. Hugh Davis and the A. H. Robins Company also consumed some women. The objects of their revenge fantasies, generally speaking, were the genitalia of Robins's executives. The cartoon in Figure 5.1 was conceived by one Dalkon

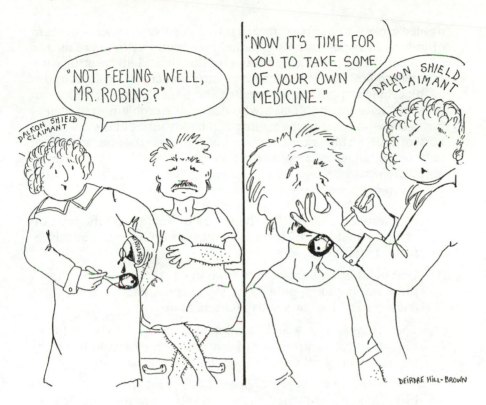

FIGURE 5.1 This cartoon epitomizes the revenge fantasies of many Dalkon Shield women. Drawn by Deirdre Hill-Brown.

Shield woman and drawn by another, an outward expression of their shared rage. The original concept for this cartoon called for a Shield to be inserted into a different orifice of Mr. Robins's body. Many other unsolicited drawings sent to DSIN were macabre in nature.

In my own case, both motives were equally important. I reflected on a sentence from my very first speech at the Richmond Rally, in July 1987: "The work I do now is for the babies I can't have but also for the healthy babies I want my daughter and all other women to be able to have."

The real challenge for DSIN activists, however, was to tap into the collective rage and yet channel it into something constructive and beneficial to the women who had been directly victimized. "I was really beginning to feel the anger of what happened to me and I needed a place to put that—to use it in a positive manner. I thought of DSIN as an opportunity to channel that energy" (Victoria Pratt).

A key theme of the group was a passionate and unwavering commitment to both maximum civil penalties and criminal prosecutions of the people responsible for creating the tragedy. Criminal prosecutions of the corporate officials who caused the problem were seen as the necessary balance to the fertility and bodily losses of these women. Loss of high public status for Robins (through the mechanism of public censure) would serve as the symbolic castration of their power; only that would be seen as equivalent to the collective loss of the victims' reproductive social status.

> Real justice would be that the family of Robins and the promoters, Dr. Hugh Davis, Lerner, and others would get life imprisonment. (Sherry Fletcher)

> First of all, I want an apology from the A. H. Robins Company. I think he should go public and say that the IUD did cause these damages and that he's sorry. (Gloria Manago)

> The Robins family should be stripped of all rights to benefit from the sale of the company, or of any money they would be receiving as a result of the shares they hold. (Victoria Pratt)

> They went into a bogus Chapter 11 . . . and we talk about this being America and what's right and this is not right and it's not fair. (Joanne Ackerman)

(It was extremely distressing to learn that the criminal investigation against Robins was dropped in January 1990, within one month of the company's merger with American Home Products [Geyelin, 1990]. No reasons were provided for dropping the charges.)

Many other women have been motivated to do something constructive with the intense anger that they feel at the betrayal perpetrated against them. Pat Cody, principal founder of DES Action, recalled the feelings that led her to question public health authorities about the early reports that DES was associated with rare vaginal cancers in daughters of women who took the drug during pregnancy.

> I got angry. It's dismissing and demeaning. It's all part of the patriarchy that makes decisions for women about their bodies. What made me so mad was that nobody was doing anything to notify people; nobody was taking responsibility. (P. Cody, personal communication, October 22, 1992).

FIRST PRIORITIES

The process of politicization is shaped by certain events, the way people interpret those events, and then how they give them political meaning (Bookman & Morgen, 1988). The first challenge for many women was how to assimilate constructively their anger and rage. DSIN did not commence with a superstructure or master plan. The first priority was to build a base of support. DSIN hoped to engage the help and support of existing organizations, presumed to be similar to our group and sympathetic to our cause. (See Chapter 4 for a detailed accounting of these attempts.) DSIN's early goals were to interrupt the dominant medical and corporate public discourse, to present a challenge to the official worldview, and to create a set of social relations where none existed before.

Although not formally recognized by the prevailing power structure as a legitimate participant in the legal negotiations, DSIN insinuated itself into the official program by carrying out its action in concert with the court's business. DSIN simply imposed itself into the litigation process. DSIN's important public events were deliberately constructed to be held during important bankruptcy court hearings. Although our opinions on important matters were not sought by the formal institutions of power, we made our demands known by holding our own press conferences. This strategy was quite successful, as the press corps was interested in a challenge to the official worldview. DSIN was perceived as a credible voice for the majority of Dalkon Shield claimants.

In the embryonic phase of this movement, an elaborate doctrine was not a high priority. A more formal organization and a complex doctrine may not have been desirable. The loose and unstructured nature of DSIN allowed the national leaders great flexibility in responding to the official court actions and Robins's legal manuvers. DSIN was both reactive (commenting on or expressing outrage about the bankruptcy court developments) and proactive (making its own demands for a worldwide recall, an FDA investigation, and criminal charges against Robins).

DIALOGUE

The primary pedagogical tool used by DSIN was dialogue. The telephone was our long-distance outreach to these isolated women. In Freire's (1985) view, dialogue is a prerequisite for radical, liberatory educa-

tion. It is a first step in consciousness raising. DSIN leaders excelled
in creating links with other Dalkon Shield women, spending long and
stressful hours listening to the harsh and sorrowful stories of others.
This is a basic feature of most self-help support groups. There is a
kind of affirmation that professionals cannot give, and this validation is empowering.

> I never knew another Dalkon Shield woman and it was very
> powerful to be able to talk to somebody who also went through
> that. Now, looking back at it, to be validated was one of the
> important experiences about it. No one else understands and
> others act condescending or hug you like a child. (Donna Reeck)

The second important step in creating an empowering dialogue
with Dalkon Shield women was to crack the legalistic rhetoric in order
to make it possible for the masses of women to have a personal stake
in the litigation. This task was not trivial. A handful of women plunged
into the difficult legalese, consulting legal allies for definitions of terms
and translations of dense and voluminous legal documents. The
women with sophisticated educational backgrounds excelled in this
role. The relevant issues had to be framed and communicated to
women in simple terms, yet without losing the vital essence. This
attempt was largely successful. DSIN's written materials (newsletters
and press statements) framed the bankruptcy litigation as a business
deal, not a program of social justice. Women became aware, through
the DSIN newsletter, that they would also have a vote on the eventual
plan of compensation and that it was in their best interests to become
educated about the complex litigation.

As individual contacts with women increased, we began to produce fact sheets as a mechanism for communicating with and educating women, as a vehicle to their empowerment, and as an alternative to the small core of volunteers spending long hours on the
telephone. (There were never more than four people who fielded the
national telephone calls, which escalated as DSIN grew.) These fact
sheets were essentially position papers. We devised a fact sheet on
the advisability of hiring a lawyer and how to negotiate with one, as
well as one analyzing the progress in the litigation, with our position on the latest developments.

Among the national leaders, dialogue, mostly in the form of a
Hegelian dialectic, was the principal means of pushing the development of an action agenda. Murdock-Vaughan and I thrashed through

most of the strategic planning, often in a confrontational manner, with each other. The heated debates and shouting matches were not hostile, however, and ultimately generated positive energy for carrying out the protest actions and other events. It was a problem-solving method that involved intense emotions and loud voices, but it was ultimately constructive and productive. In an interview for this book, Cinders Murdock-Vaughan recalled this dialectic among leaders:

> In my experience with problem solving, yelling had always been really negative. This brought a sort of intellectual bantering into my life that had been lacking. I realized that we could fight, we could disagree, and it would still be okay. It didn't mean the organization was going to fall apart. It was a kind of intellectual tool that I learned. That was an important realization for me to come to, and once I had that, I felt much freer to argue sometimes for the sake of argument . . . that was just part of the process we went through.

The plan for the next DSIN move was often made at the conclusion of a previous event, with several DSIN leaders or members who had participated in the event planning the next move. During the period of greatest activism, there were rarely more than four people (not always the same four people) shaping the public action events. As we made more contacts, Murdock-Vaughan, Reeck, some of the chapter leaders, and I all consulted with many parties, including lawyers and other public interest groups, depending on the issue at hand. The process, as it evolved, was always more important than the development of a complex group doctrine or structure; that is, we were always flying by the seat of our pants.

DSIN LEADERSHIP PROFILE

The women who committed to DSIN leadership felt passionately about the issues of injustice and justice. The compensation settlement being negotiated in the Richmond court was not the motivating factor in their commitment to activism. Their energy was fueled by their anger and rage for their grave physical injuries and by their elation at relief from aloneness. The variety of personal goals and commitments among DSIN leaders included (1) retribution against A. H. Robins for the reckless violation of women's bodies and the loss of fertility; (2)

an urgent need to communicate the facts about the tragedy to the general public, from the survivors' perspective; and (3) a desire to help other victims to feel supported and validated.

> I wanted to try to make a difference. I felt Robins was getting away with what they would call the perfect crime. I had no idea of what was involved, but when I found out that they had destroyed records, then I wanted to try to help people who were in the same position that I was. (Joanne Ackerman)

> I wish I could have afforded to take out a full-page ad or rented billboards on the highway. I would have done that if that's what it would have taken to educate people. (Sherry Fletcher)

During the course of three years, 28 women volunteered to become chapter coordinators in their local areas. The women represented a broad cross-section of the general population. More than 50% of them had some college education. Three of them were pursuing college degrees during their DSIN activism. Four of the leaders were African-Americans. There were chapters in every major geographical region of the United States. There was no real concentration of chapters in any one geographical region, although Pennsylvania (the home state of the national office) did have three chapters.

There may be a correlation between the degree of commitment to and participation in this particular political fight and the degree of the injury that women suffered. All the leaders interviewed for this book described their injuries as life-altering. This meant variously that they were unable to have children, had endured divorce, had experienced severe financial hardships related to the complications of their injuries, or a combination of these factors. More than 80% of the leaders had experienced at least one divorce. All attribute their marital strains to the infertility and health problems caused by the Dalkon Shield.

> I hadn't been married even a year. I was a young woman, 22 years old, just been married, and I had this horrible operation in my abdomen. I was sore; it hurt. I had 24 wire sutures put inside me that hurt all the time for 8 years . . . so sex wasn't the most wonderful thing in the world. I was a newlywed! It hurt to have sex. (Fran Cleary)

> I will never have the health I had before. I take 2 milligrams of estrogen every day. There have been problems. I have not been

interested in things that I might have been. Maybe it's the depression. (Shirley Nichols)

It changed my home, my family, my husband. It was like 360 degrees—a whole circle that came about. (Gloria Manago)

Generally, the women who committed to DSIN leadership were more informed than the average Dalkon Shield victim and were eager to have as much information as they could get. They describe themselves as independent, self-reliant, and persistent. Many of them characterize themselves as fighters. There was a general feeling that *somebody* had to wage this fight, and they wanted to be part of it. Although they were political amateurs, the women interviewed for this book all spoke of the collective leadership as the most important resource of the organization. "We have put in our blood and guts. We've lived it and breathed it, lived it and died it" (Sherry Fletcher).

Approximately 50% of DSIN leaders had had previous community organizing experience—for example, in Girl Scouts, Planned Parenthood, and church groups. However, none of the women interviewed for this research described themselves as having had prior *political* experience, and they did not think of themselves as "politicians" in a classical or traditional sense. To be a real politician, they all felt, you have to run a campaign to be elected to a formal position in a formal institution of power.

When I first founded DSIN, I remember trying to contact Lois Gibbs, a former blue-collar housewife who waged the Love Canal environmental fight. Her original energies resulted in a major community protest, in the 1970s, against the Hooker Chemical Company, which had buried toxic wastes underneath her suburban housing development in upstate New York (Levine, 1982). I knew that she had achieved a remarkable degree of success in conducting a grass-roots campaign. Gibbs has been successful in moving beyond the embryonic stage of a protest movement and is today widely acknowledged as an important leader in the environmental movement. Today Gibbs is the executive director of the Environmental Justice Center, coordinating more than 7,000 grass-roots groups. In a recent newsletter published by her organization, she offered some observations on the characteristics of women in the environmental movement:

> Although these women come from a variety of backgrounds, most are not trained organizers, political strategists, or business managers but are moms, full time homemakers, family farmers, or other workers. They would not categorize themselves as warriors, yet that is exactly what

they are. These women are fearless, determined, courageous, and unwilling to compromise when the issue is health and safety for their families, their communities, and the environment. (Gibbs, 1992, p. 2)

Although I believe Gibbs's description is flattering and accurate, "determined" strikes me as a serious understatement of Dalton Shield leaders' level of involvement and commitment. My own determination to work on this cause became obsessive behavior. I worked at least 16 hours a day for several years. I believe that certain aspects of my personality, namely those of being an academic overachiever and a perfectionist, explain both the strengths and the weaknesses that came to characterize my participation in this cause. Other leaders also report being overinvolved. One chapter leader characterized her own behavior as "PID on the brain." Reeck did a superhuman job of fielding telephone calls, sometimes talking to as many as 50 women in a single day.

I couldn't not answer the telephone. I couldn't reject talking to a woman and saying "Yeah, I know what it's like." It was addictive to feel that powerful to be able to help people heal, to take away their blame and guilt. It was better than sex. (Donna Reeck)

In order for movements to move beyond the embryonic stage, it is necessary for the participants to work through this problem, if it exists. To prevent the great potential for burnout, leaders should achieve an overt awareness of their personal limitations and adopt a healthy sense of balance between their commitment to the "cause" and their personal lives.

On the other hand, the intensity of commitment and participation can be positive, exciting, and transforming. The planning of a course of political action, and watching how it unfolds, can be a rewarding challenge. Being bold and taking risks can create a type of euphoria. Highly charged public displays produce a visceral, physical "high." The immediacy of the events demands quick action. Before the Nike sportshoe ad appeared, we were living by the motto "Just do it!"

If it is possible to think of compulsive behavior as positive in any way, I would say that such single-minded "determination" on the part of a small number of people, who harness and channel their energies toward a positive goal, can be a powerful force. The most precious resources of social protest groups are the personal passions, commitments, and energies of their members. Remarkable social reform can be accomplished, or at least initiated, with very few people.

I must also address the "courageous" quality that Gibbs attributes to women leaders of social movements. When carrying out DSIN's public protest events, I was terrified most of the time: I did not think of myself as courageous. I was the one person, at the national level, whose hometown and home telephone number circulated widely. Three factors fueled me to push ahead despite my personal fears: (1) every time I heard another story of grotesque injury and medical mistreatment, I got angrier; (2) the negative experiences with some of our legal "advocates" and the rumors of the judge's bias in favor of the Robins Company enraged me; and (3) injured women who could not themselves go public encouraged all of us to keep up the good fight.

I was not the only one who felt fear. After a number of us were actively leading this protest movement, we shared our fears with each other and dubbed the phenomenon "the Silkwood syndrome." (See the section entitled "Confronting the System" in Chapter 3.) Gibbs (1992) does make a conclusion that is corroborated by all the DSIN leaders: "Our opponents have not yet figured out that intimidation and violence doesn't work against women, it only makes us more determined and willing to go that extra mile to win" (p. 2).

Developing the Leadership

Chapter leaders were first recruited from participants at the Richmond Rally in July 1987 and from the group of women who contacted DSIN in the first year of its existence. It is a great challenge and risk for an organization to develop leaders from a random population of women, as DSIN did. (In contrast, NOW had been founded by a select group of women [Davis, 1991]). There was no application or review process, and there were no criteria applied of chapter leaders, except that they be willing to fund their own local activities. Most of these commitments were made over the telephone by women who had never met each other. A detailed, written instruction kit on how to organize a chapter was devised and sent to each chapter leader.

About six of the chapter leaders initiated frequent contact with the national leaders, but, except for one face-to-face meeting at the Richmond conference in February 1988 and several public meetings (in Maryland, North Carolina, and Los Angeles), DSIN business was conducted primarily by telephone and mail. Small groups of DSIN members met one another in Richmond from time to time for court hearings, and everyone who showed up there helped to plan future DSIN events.

Communications originated with the national leaders and spread outward to the chapter leaders. The majority of the frequent mailings were informational items about the status of the negotiations or DSIN's organizational response to important events or issues as they developed. The goal of these mailings was to empower the chapter leaders to frame their own responses to those events in their local media or with their local contacts. Items that chapter leaders sent in or articles they researched were also circulated to all leaders. Press releases prepared by DSIN national leaders were sent to them for distribution in their regions. When possible, the press releases were customized to include the names of the local chapter leaders in order to facilitate local coverage.

The 1988 Richmond conference, attended by about 20 chapter leaders, was important to the continuing commitment of the chapter leaders to the cause. This meeting was an example of what DSIN needed in order to grow and thrive. It provided important bonding among the leaders:

> The Richmond conference changed my life, and I mean that. I've had a pretty exciting life but that experience stands out in my mind as the one opportunity I've had as an individual and as a member of something larger, to really feel the loss. . . . I was overwhelmed by the enormity of it. I could look around me at a group of women who were *real*. (Victoria Pratt)

> That really bonded us. That really made me feel a part of the group. That's why I still feel close, in spite of the long distance. (Shirley Nichols)

DSIN Power Structure

In order to create the appearance that DSIN was larger and more organized than it was, I adopted the title of president to describe my national leadership role. As sole founder and president of DSIN during the first year of its existence, I continued to retain the largest share of power after Murdock-Vaughan became vice-president and Reeck became secretary. I maintained the files and records, initiated most of the external contacts and negotiations, wrote most of the group's documents, handled most of the arrangements for press conferences, and served as the chief spokesperson. Murdock-Vaughan collaborated with me on many related projects, managed a large share of the telephone support work, spoke with many of the lawyers involved in the case, and eventually assumed major responsibilities for press conferences and chapter coordination. Reeck gradually increased her activism: She began by coordinating most of the mass mailings, eventually handled most of the telephone support work, traveled with Murdock-Vaughan and me to many Richmond Court hearings, and represented DSIN on projects with allied organizations.

In terms of our personal strengths, as an educator I had the most professionally relevant employment experience for articulating the philosophy and goals of the group and for developing the written documents. As a university administrator of a large research institute, I had acquired management skills that helped DSIN get organized. Murdock-Vaughan and Reeck both excelled in developing and maintaining interpersonal relationships. This combination of talents enhanced the group's accomplishments.

DSIN Power Issue

My unilateral decision not to move ahead with the coalition (described in Chapter 4) dramatized an internal hierarchy in the relationships among the three national leaders. Murdock-Vaughan was frustrated by my decision but did not confront me at the time. She expressed her real feelings by talking to Reeck and by writing in a diary. She shared some of her writings in the context of an interview for this book. The following excerpt of a letter she wrote to me, but never mailed, also points to the difficulty we had in confronting each other directly when conflicts arose:

> Your unilateral decision [not to join the coalition] seems to have been made from a purely personal standpoint. Why wasn't there more input from individuals who have spent almost as much time and energy as you have? Why weren't alternatives, such as delegating authority among those willing to take it, explored? Why don't we empower the chapter heads on this? Why don't you trust your own strengths more to affect the outcome? Why don't you take the advice of more experienced women on this?

In the interview for this book, Murdock-Vaughan situates herself in what she calls a "supporting role" in regard to leadership. She always saw herself as subordinate in the leadership power structure.

Although it did not lead to fragmentation of the organization, this episode involving the coalition did begin to dissipate her personal investment in DSIN. Reeck also was disappointed. She no longer felt as empowered or as enthusiastic about persevering with the long-term goals of the group.

After the stresses of the coalition episode, the three of us agreed to a change in the leadership structure. We became co-chairs and negotiated the division of labor. We began to hold more frequent telephone conference calls to discuss DSIN business and make strategic decisions. Both Reeck and Murdock-Vaughan believed, however, that maintaining our friendship and bonds with one another was more important than fragmenting DSIN and moving out on their own. In retrospect, they also agree that after this episode, enthusiasm for the long-term goals began to wane. For my part, I felt conflicted by the results of this event; I was quite burned out, and my own enthusiasm also began to diminish. In spite of these problems, the three of us persevered as a team for another year of intense participation.

By December 1988, Murdock-Vaughan, Thompson, Reeck, and I acknowledged that our patterns of involvement resembled addictive behavior. This frightened us, and we vowed to withdraw somewhat and to monitor one another in order to restore some sense of balance in our lives. I have memories of going through a withdrawal process during December 1988 and January 1989: I was physically ill most of this time. I ceased most of my DSIN activities and rarely talked to anyone about the case. For the next year and a half, my involvement in Dalkon Shield–related activities tended to be a matter of "all-or-nothing."

TRASHING AND FRAGMENTATION

The general literature on social movements includes reports of factionalism and fragmentation occurring within social protest movements (Levine, 1982; Wilson, 1973). Blumberg and West (1989) speak of the fusion and fission of groups, regardless of gender, as "an important and frequent process in the rise and fall of social movements" (p. 9). Most social movements spend as much time and energy fighting one another as they do the common enemy, according to Levine. This problem is not confined to cases of women organizing.

The problems of internal hierarchies in women's groups are also common, even in feminist organizations that have made deliberate, ideological commitments to democratic and egalitarian power structures. Davis (1991), Carden (1974), Freeman (1975), and Ruzek (1978) address the problems of schisms and dissension in women's movement organizations. Unequal power distribution has often created strain within women's liberation groups (Ruzek, 1978).

The fact that factions develop is not troublesome. The problem is the lack of experience that women have in facing conflict and hostility and in dealing openly with confrontation in a constructive or productive manner. Women need to develop skills that will allow them to manage contentious intergroup and intragroup relations. In the overall scheme of a social movement, every group makes an important contribution in its own way. It is far better for noncooperating groups to coexist than it is for any group's energies to be diverted toward defeating another group. It is simply unproductive and self-defeating to waste precious time and energy on intergroup hostility, because the negative energies spent on this benefit the common enemy.

The feminist literature reports that conflict resolution in the women's movement includes character assassination (called *trashing*) when tensions arise among women (Joreen, 1976). MacPherson (1986) discusses trashing that occurred during the evolution of a feminist self-help group called The Menopause Collective. She is inspired to be brutally honest about the conflicts and contradictions because such conflict is not a trivial issue in the process of women's organizing around an issue of social injustice. The Menopause Collective was torn by internal difficulties, including competition among and demeaning of members.

> It is disappointing to recognize that while feminists, by definition, are in conflict with men in a patriarchal society, we are also in internal conflict within our own feminist organizations because of our differences. (MacPherson, 1986, p. 55)

MacPherson offers a solution. Women should learn to protect one another in their contradictions, and feminists, like others, must learn to appreciate the diversity of women's interests and needs. Diversity does not have to mean divisiveness, however. Criticism, in the context of love and concern for one another, can be action toward transformation, which strengthens each individual and group. Although I concur with MacPherson's sentiments, I believe that her solution is idealistic and I am not optimistic that this approach is realistic. The single-mindedness of leaders totally committed to their organizations makes it difficult for them to extend goodwill in this fashion. It is far preferable for group members to part company and retain respect for their counterparts. Fission can be productive if people have reached the point of becoming ineffective because of their differences.

Gender socialization may be a contributing factor to the existence of this problem. Girls are socialized to be quiet, agreeable, and focused on maintaining pleasant social relations. When conflict erupts during play, girls typically cry and sulk, go home, or deprecate their opponents. Likewise, the socialization process pressures girls toward the cultural ideal of affiliation with one another, which makes it difficult for girls to rise above the crowd and assume leadership roles. That privilege is typically reserved for boys. This may translate to a negative valuation of women who do become leaders. Phrases such as "power hungry" and "just making a name for herself" are commonly used by some women to describe women who assume leadership roles in adulthood. This was one dimension of inner conflict that I experienced as a leader; I was fearful of such criticism from others.

The socialization pressures on boys are reversed. The conditioning of males to stand up to the rigors and challenges of political life begins early, perhaps as early as the school playground and the Little League baseball field. Childhood games are a training ground for the public arena of politics. Adversarial relations and conflict resolution are ritualized into boys' games and sporting events. Girls play few games with elaborate rules or organization. The rules of boys' games are expected to be hotly contested, and an openly confrontational, competitive, and aggressive manner characterizes that play.

DSIN leaders were fascinated with the Richmond courtroom behavior of lawyers. It appeared outwardly to us that the men involved in the official proceedings were desensitized to the anger and confrontational style that characterized their relations during the court hearings. Lawyers on both sides of the room appeared to us to direct hostility toward one another. We took their emotional outbursts and searing comments to one another at face value, and we were made uncomfortable by them. Then, at the end of the day, these same lawyers would chat amiably with one another outside the courtroom and, in some cases, would even go out to dinner or socialize with one another.

Political inexperience and naiveté is a partial explanation for the seriousness with which we responded to confrontation, and conformity to gender-appropriate behavior may explain why we engage in avoidance behavior on many occasions involving conflict. I concur with both Carden (1974) and Freeman (1975) that the better approach to this problem is for differing groups to adopt some strategy of "agreeing to disagree" with one another. However, reaching that understanding and adhering to it are not easy or natural. Movement leaders who are engaged in obsessive, passionate commitments will be defensive and narrowly focused on their viewpoints, thus finding it difficult to compromise.

Training programs for community activists and other such programs should address this dynamic head-on. Better yet would be more practical experience with conflict resolution for children of both genders, through the medium of play. I do not wish to glorify the current system of competition that characterizes boys' games and men's adult political gaming. In the adult political arena, more than one man has been assassinated (literally) by his opponents. I suggest that training and conscious awareness are required to learn how to manage the inevitability of conflict in a healthy way. Adults of both genders also need this training.

When product-liability reform battles rage in the U.S. Congress, the Ralph Nader organizations have been successful in rallying victims' groups to lobby against big business. So far, the legislative initiatives backed by major corporations on this issue have been defeated every year. The consumer movement has been successful in mobilizing disparate single-issue organizations. An analogous coordination of efforts and collaboration on legislation or political pressure to draw attention to women's health issues would produce better results than we have so far seen in reforming women's health. At the present time, however, there is no all-embracing alliance or mechanism for bringing different groups together.

OTHER DALKON SHIELD WOMEN

Only a small number of all the women who contacted DSIN actually supported the cause, either by joining the organization, sending us letters of encouragement, or becoming leaders. In the final analysis, DSIN had at least one contact with more than 20,000 Dalkon Shield users. Merely belonging to an oppressed group does not ensure individual consciousness of inequity or a willingness to fight.

Victim-blaming ideologies make it difficult for victims to generate a collective consciousness, and victims often contribute to the maintenance of their own victimization (Kidder and Fine, 1986). DSIN leaders were always skeptical about the hidden agendas of others, and some women were also skeptical of DSIN. Some women with high expectations of large monetary awards were fearful that DSIN activities could jeopardize their settlements. Several women called me in anger, rebuking me personally for this possibility. Other women reported that their lawyers had instructed them not to contact DSIN.

Several DSIN chapter leaders had followed DSIN activities through the newspapers for some time before contacting the organization. Many women mentioned a deep-seated suspicion for anyone in the public forum. The Dalkon Shield case created circumstances ripe for further victimization, and the feelings of vulnerability run deep in this population:

> I have a real fear about being exploited. I don't want to be exploited by lawyers. I have been exploited by A. H. Robins. I don't want to be exploited by any group. I know you're not someone who is just trying to make a name for yourself, or that is trying to exploit us. If I had not gone to the Richmond conference, then in my mind I would have been fearful. I would have wondered what the real reason for DSIN was—what connections the group had. (Shirley Nichols)

Even among a geographically intact population such as the Love Canal residents, there were different subgroups and suspicions. The residents held different belief systems, perceived the problems differently, and acted differently depending on their age, the location of their home, and whether they owned or rented. The same is true of the Dalkon Shield population. Besides their geographical dispersion, significant differences among these women included the nature and severity of the injuries, age, marital status, life goals, long-term versus minor sequelae, socioeconomic status (particularly as it related to health care access), employment, and religious affiliation.

A major reason for lack of engagement was psychological. Post-traumatic stress disorder (PTSD), much discussed and written about in the 1970s by mental health professionals working with Vietnam veterans (Figley, 1985), can affect people who survive life-threatening injuries such as those from the Dalkon Shield. Many Dalkon Shield survivors found self-affirmation through applying descriptions of PTSD to some of their own psychic and emotional states. Many women reported experiencing severe distress when thinking about the circumstance that created their injuries ("flashbacks"), and all kinds of everyday stimuli may have triggered intense stress reactions, for example, going to a baby shower for a pregnant woman.

> When I talk to women, they're very excited to hear that we're out here, and then I don't hear from them again . . . because all the things that they're learning brings it all back and makes it very hard. . . . It's sort of debilitating in a way. They live it over again, they feel so helpless and victimized and finding out all the details can be unnerving. (Jan Thompson)

One woman gave up her activism with the group because of the personal distress it caused. "I wish that I could have psychologically handled it but it was too defeating for me" (Joanne Ackerman).

THE IMPACT OF RACE AND SOCIAL CLASS

Social-class status is a relevant factor in women's leadership and active participation in a social movement. More than 90% of DSIN leaders could be categorized as being middle-middle to upper-middle class. They knew they would have to fund their local activities. They were social workers, schoolteachers, hairdressers, women not employed outside the home, factory workers, fitness instructors, and secretaries. Several women were permanently disabled and unemployed due to their Dalkon Shield–related complications.

Social class and ethnic differences have been a serious problem for health activists, according to Ruzek. Middle-class women dominate the organized groups. These women are more likely to have the personal economic resources to participate in such social movements, which are inherently volunteer in nature. Although we did maintain good relations with individual women from different class and ethnic backgrounds, it was difficult to engage women who were not of European background as leaders.

Of the twenty-eight DSIN leaders, four were African-American. Of these four, only one managed to develop a highly visible and extremely active local chapter. Although the other three women clearly felt invested in DSIN, the fourth woman was the most effective leader. She also had the highest socioeconomic status and educational level of the four and a background as a professional social worker, which contributed to her ability to organize around this issue. In fact, this woman led the largest DSIN chapter. Most of the women who participated in this chapter were also African-American. In general, however, most of the DSIN leaders were Caucasian, middle-class women.

FUNDING

With a cause identified as women's special responsibility, female reformers are able to maintain leadership and direct the action. The benefits of such poltical independence, however, are often tempered by a corresponding lack of financial resources, a major impediment that plagued DSIN.

The volunteer aspect of social movements may have some gender specificity. Women's grass-roots organizations are often labeled *kitchen-table operations* because they are first organized in informal ways, with few financial or material resources. The positive dimension of this imagery is that women can stay at home and maintain some semblance of a personal life. For example, DSIN leaders cooked meals and folded laundry while conducting DSIN business on the telephone. However, the fact that women's contributions to social movements are volunteer means they assume these responsibilities in addition to one or perhaps two other full-time jobs—paid employment and family obligations.

Social scientists have drawn ample attention to the fact that women's labor is already undervalued, both politically and economically. DSIN leaders never put a price tag on their labor and never received any type of compensation for their work. In an analysis of the civil rights movement, Blumberg and West (1989) observed that, when the movement gained a measure of success and growth, men took over the leadership roles and the formal, paid positions. This is reminiscent of the male Dalkon Shield lawyer from Group B, who seemed to me to have too much control over that group's function. He had also orchestrated his group's plans for the coalition press conference that had been a pivotal moment in DSIN's life, too (see detailed discussion in Chapter 4).

Grass-roots groups are caught in a bind. In order to generate funding from outsiders, they must offer proof of their ability to accomplish worthwhile goals. On the other hand, they need funds in order to implement activities. Some foundations understand this dilemma and have special "seed" funding categories; our first appeals to feminist organizations in these categories were turned down because all funds for reproductive rights issues were going to grass-roots groups engaged in the abortion battle.

Our first public event (the Richmond rally) was funded primarily by our personal funds. Printed materials that we generated for that rally and media coverage of the event were helpful for developing grant proposals. DSIN received two modest grants from the Civil Justice Foundation in October 1987, which supported various press conferences and the expenses of the Richmond conference in February 1988. A group called Lawyers for Consumer Rights, a nonprofit organization based in Harrisburg, Pennsylvania, printed and mailed several issues of our newsletter, which would not otherwise have been possible. Other than that, DSIN has relied totally on voluntary donations, which were modest and undependable. DSIN has always had a deficit, and leaders have covered the shortages with personal outlays for traveling and phone bills. DSIN developed a mandate for greater activism as the group blossomed, but it was short on resources to implement action. The lack of substantive financial resources and the geographical distances between members also hindered DSIN's ability to institutionalize and continue. Wilson (1973) addresses this problem as a general one plaguing social movements: "A wider review of monographs in the field reveals that most social movmements are impoverished, operating with hopelessly inadequate resources most of the time" (p. 168).

Possible explanations for this severe funding problem are:

1. Nobody in DSIN had enough expertise to perform serious development work or to persist in fundraising against great odds and a staggering work load.
2. The particular historical era had hundreds of fine social causes competing for severely limited funds.
3. The cause was too narrow or too controversial for most foundations, which have substantial corporate participation.

Of these possibilities, the first was certainly true. About four different chapter leaders attempted to write proposals and find sponsors. No one ever volunteered to specialize in this role. The second reason is plausible, since DSIN eventually applied to the Ms. Foundation and received encouragement; however, the resurgence of the threat to abortion rights preempted that organization's allocations to other worthy reproductive rights issues. The third is also plausible, since the source of the Dalkon Shield problem was identifiable—nameable corporate executives.

In spite of funding problems, DSIN achieved an extraordinary degree of activism and success with the limited resources it did have.

DSIN's expenditures in three years totaled around $34,000. This does not count all the chapter leaders' personal expenditures, nor were there ever any paid salaries. A dollar value on all the women's labor costs has never been factored in.

MEDIA POWER

Media publicity is increasingly popular, especially for poor and powerless groups that cannot afford expensive legal or lobbying strategies (Wolfsfeld, 1990). The mass media are a gateway to power, particularly when formal institutions ignore the powerless.

> Political movements must rely on large-scale communications in order to *matter* but in the process, they become newsworthy only by submitting to the implicit rules of newsmaking, by conforming to journalistic notions of what a "story" is, what an "event" is, what a "protest" is. The processed image then tends to *become* the movement for wider audiences (Gitlin, 1990, p. 276).

The risk in attracting media attention, however, is in not being portrayed the way the group desires in order for it to be positioned as powerful in some way. The mass media have the power to define the public significance of a movement. By covering movement events, they lend legitimacy; by ignoring them, they deprive them of larger significance (Gitlin, 1990). This delicate situation led DSIN leaders into lengthy discussions about how to identify the group and goals to the outside world in a positive way.

The following observations reflect the direct experience that DSIN leaders had with the press. Social relations between system challengers and the media must be conducted as deliberately and carefully as those of any corporate public relations department. Patience, diplomacy, and skill with press contacts are vital to any protest group's success in gaining a forum in the mass media. No matter how insensitive reporters are, spokespersons for opposition groups cannot afford to offend them. The media validate a cause, certify spokespersons on social issues, and create personalities.

Press and media people are conduits of information. The reporters talk to many parties—almost every important player in the game. They may pass along messages between allies or even antagonists, or ask questions that the challenger may not have an opportunity to ask directly of the stakeholders in the formal institutions.

Reporters must be educated about issues before they will cover the story. The compelling aspects of the issue must be framed for them. Once they understand that there is a story to be had, however, publications compete with one another to break a story. Giving the highest-status publication an exclusive hot tip can lead to some form of reciprocity—information not available directly from the authorities, for instance.

Certain types of publications or divisions within major newspapers are interested in a narrow aspect of any given issue, which means that a group's social relations involve reporters with different perspectives who raise different questions. Reporters can also decide to cover particular dimensions of and perspectives on an issue that they themselves are interested in or biased toward. They regularly formulate their own hypotheses about an issue and then test them out through a semistructured interview format with various informants. They are fairly interested in conflict or opposition, although being interviewed as the challenger guarantees neither mention in an article nor the type of mention that one would desire. Different publications tend to certify particular authorities or personalities and return to them repeatedly for comment.

News about the Dalkon Shield case appeared only on the financial pages of major urban newspapers before the public protest actions of DSIN began. In an attempt to change this, DSIN courted the media, although no one in the group had previous media experience. Early assistance from a university media specialist was invaluable in constructing professional-looking press advisories and press kits. Press advisories should also be sent by the challengers to all parties central to the case who should know that there are protest plans in the works.

All printed press releases were carefully crafted in the most simple terms, attempting to convey only one or two major ideas, yet presenting DSIN as the challenger to the official worldview. The verbal anger was aimed at A. H. Robins, not the court. Themes reflected the betrayal of trust, the loss of reproductive capacities, and anticipation that justice would be served. Some quotes from chapter leaders at a November 1987 press conference frame the messages:

Let's shatter the myth that Robins is bankrupt. Their profit margin is higher than ever and women continue to suffer.

I think it's terrible that they used us as guinea pigs.

It's like a holocaust. They led people blindly. Masses of women were taken to destruction.

The rhetoric also involved deliberate decisions about whether to refer to ourselves in the media as *victims* or *survivors*. Some of our advisors and consultants encouraged us to use the term *victim*. As our empowerment as leaders grew, however, those of us who acted as spokespersons wanted to use the term *survivor* to give other Dalkon Shield women hope and courage about transforming themselves into empowered women also. There were a variety of feelings about this among DSIN leaders. In the end, we all used a different approach and we tried to address the use of these terms at a conscious level with reporters, with mixed results.

> What I have found is that *victim* tends to get the attention of the media faster, and at first, I didn't like that. Then I decided that if that's what it takes to get the message across, it doesn't matter what they call me. On a personal level, I like to think of myself as a survivor because I don't play the victim role. (Victoria Pratt)

> I think it's been very detrimental to us to have been labeled *victims*. When women hear that, they identify with being a victim, and they feel helpless and a lot of women feel like there's nothing they can do. (Jan Thompson)

> I want women to have pride and not shame. When I talked to women on the phone, you could see how using the word *survivor* would adjust their mindset about themselves. I always tried to project that they were lucky, that they've overcome this through their strength. (Donna Reeck)

Many women who contacted DSIN tried fervently to get this issue covered on the daytime television talk shows, which are so widely broadcast. Many "women's problems" have been disclosed through that medium. Oprah Winfrey received many appeals from Dalkon Shield women to do a show on the subject, including several attempts by DSIN. We provided her producers with most of the excellent printed materials available on the Shield. Other groups and individuals also tried, to no avail. We received no explanation. None of the other famous talk show hosts wanted to do a show, either. The "Phil Donahue Show" declined, saying that they had covered the issue once, years ago, and that the issue was now "dead." The topic is as sad and gruesome as any other that they do cover. The lack of coverage of this issue must involve the commercial realities of the major television networks. The pharmaceutical industry is a major advertiser on these shows, and the targets of our rage were identifiable corporate executives in pharmaceutical companies. These daytime talk shows rarely, if ever, do programs where corporate blame can be fixed. The "MacNeil-Lehrer Newshour" was the only national television program to air a major report on the case, a 1988 segment that included a favorable and comprehensive profile of the women's perspective.

Given DSIN's limited resources and lack of experience, the group was quite successful in gaining media coverage. First, DSIN prepared a deliberate and careful set of background materials that the press accepted as valid and reliable. Reporters do not want to research background, particularly on an issue as complex as the Dalkon Shield case. DSIN sent a coherent, valid history of the case and the group in response to every press inquiry. The organization also served as a referral service for the media to experts and other stakeholders on almost every aspect of the case. DSIN became indispensable to some of the reporters, who cultivated us for our ability to provide information and referrals to other parties, saving them time preparing articles for publication. Second, DSIN members who worked on press releases were articulate, writing them in simple, nonlegal language that could distill the complexity of the case without losing the vital essence of the issues.

Holding press conferences at the National Press Club in Washington, D.C., was a deliberate tactic; the site has an aura of legitimacy, and the press corps, naturally, congregate there. Murdock-Vaughan and I concluded this from tracking other national news stories and gleaning bits of information from successful press conferences by watching television news shows and participating in press conferences sponsored by Ralph Nader. We also learned that it was important to stage press conferences with deliberation—that is, to make the most effective use of props and visuals and to properly position spokespersons.

We had learned by this time that a pack of reporters tracks any given story and will usually follow major events associated with it. We could not afford a clipping service, but by reading a variety of national newspapers we were able to build a large media mailing list from the bylines on Dalkon Shield stories. Our own press releases were mailed to all those people, even if we had not had previous personal contact with them.

In retrospect, it seems probable that DSIN's basic success in being presented by the media in a positive light was due to the fact that the concerns and values of this social movement coincided with the concerns and values of elites in both politics and the media (Gitlin, 1990). The DSIN protest was aimed not at destroying the system but

at inducing the formal institutions to act on their stated ideals and
to respond to the violation of women's socially sanctioned right to
reproduce.

SUCCESSES

In the short space of three years, DSIN conducted the following activities simultaneously with only a handful of people, none of whom had
ever led such efforts before:

• Outreach and networking to approximately 40 different existing
  organizations, educating them about who Dalkon Shield women
  were and soliciting their assistance and support on various issues
• Multiple attempts at locating sympathetic funding agencies and
  writing grant proposals
• Building the collective and communicating with neophyte chapter
  leaders and thousands of other Dalkon Shield users on the telephone
• Learning how to conduct a media campaign, including preparing
  professional-looking press releases and press kits, organizing approximately 10 major press conferences, and appearing on national and
  regional television shows
• Generating and mailing a massive volume of written materials, such
  as fact sheets on various topics, individual correspondence, and
  guidelines for chapter development
• Forming and maintaining relations with numerous lawyers and
  other groups who were direct participants in the Dalkon Shield case,
  whom we consulted in order to plan our next moves
• Conducting the public "fight" by attending major court hearings
  in Richmond and protesting outside the courthouse
• Attending and participating in numerous events sponsored by allied
  organizations, mostly related to product liability or corporate
  responsibility or both.

The success or failure of any movement is only part of the story
of empowerment. The changes and transformations of the women
who participate in collective actions are important: "Their empowerment is visible in the transformations of their views of themselves as
women and in their capacity to understand and change the world they
live in" (Bookman & Morgen, 1988, p. 19). DSIN women interviewed

for this research expressed a variety of ways in which they were empowered by their engagement in this cause.

> Now I'm involved in the fight against tort reform in Wisconsin, and I get a sense through that that we can do something. I am fighting for corporate responsibility, and that's confronting the beast and I do like confronting that beast. (Victoria Pratt)

> First, it was wonderful to meet some other women and be validated. Then, I realized there was a hunger for something else. I started taking the phone calls, but not for a personal need anymore, but to try to impart some of the peace I found for myself and some of the political workings. There's nothing that's been a more powerful experience than this in my life. (Donna Reeck)

As a result of their involvement in this social movement, many DSIN leaders are doing things now that they had not done previously. Donna Reeck registered to vote for the first time in her life because she realized one person *can* make a difference. Shirley Nichols had the confidence to handle her own claim rather than hire a lawyer. Jan Thompson is applying to law school and writing a proposal to create a legal clinic for Dalkon Shield claimants. Victoria Pratt is becoming involved in community leadership organizations at the national level.

DSIN leaders attribute the organization's successes to a wide variety of factors. Most of the women interviewed for this research spoke with pride about the most precious resource we had—the leaders of the group. "We've all fallen prey to this dishonest corporate tactic, and the impact it's had on us as individuals is what gives us our strength, and in turn, will give the organization its strength" (Victoria Pratt).

Another important factor in our success is that this organization gained considerable legitimacy with many parties. We were able, in spite of a limited number of leaders, to attend to multiple constituents—from other injured women, to the judge and the press, to other public interest allies. We were a group of amateurs who filled a necessary niche. We were able to articulate the needs of a wide range of women. We were not identified with any special-interest group.

Finally, we adopted a deliberate strategy of rational tactics as opposed to brash guerrilla-theater tactics, which might have gotten us portrayed as hysterical women and, thus, discounted. Although bizarre visual images could have been presented—some women, for example, fantasized about pushing empty baby carriages draped in black—we deliberately avoided such sensational or "radical" tactics. DSIN did not want to be portrayed like Students for a Democratic Society (SDS), the bra-burning feminists (an unfair and distorted image feminists suffered from for years), or such anti-choice groups as Operation Rescue. The most radical visual aid DSIN used during the protest actions in Richmond was deliberately wearing black clothing with large, white paper Dalkon Shields pinned to the shoulders. Many women even wore those Shields into the courtroom. A Richmond television newscaster once focused on the Shields, referring to them as our "badge of honor." Additionally, the women of the Los Angeles chapter adopted a uniform of sorts for chapter meetings, always wearing red and black to symbolize the blood and death associated with the Shield.

LIMITATIONS

Understanding reasons for organizational weakness contributes to future gains and victories in the politicization process. DSIN did not achieve cohesiveness of its disparate and isolated membership. No Dalkon Shield group achieved this goal. The reasons for this are unclear, but some of the contributing factors discussed in this book include wide geographical dispersion, blind trust in the official institutions of power, the false notion that unity was possible, and the fact that there was a compensation program. The last reason moderated many claimants' involvement so as not to jeopardize their financial settlements.

The fact that communication within DSIN consisted mainly of long-distance telephone relationships hindered its growth and effectiveness as a political pressure group, and this in turn hampered the group's ability to move beyond the embryonic phase of a social movement and on to the construction of a more institutionalized organization. There were not enough continuous, face-to-face meetings to work out a group doctrine, and there was no real forum or mechanism either for addressing and resolving internal differences or conflicts or for formulating long-term organizational strategy.

The mostly long-distance relationships hindered the speed with which we reached positions, did not provide a real opportunity to work out an elaborate doctrine or even to address and resolve conflict among ourselves as a group, and kept us at the level of a loosely connected network rather than a more formal institution.

The small number of people involved meant they were overtaxed and almost inevitably led to a burnout problem.

SUMMARY

The traditional definition of power as domination over others explains the limited success of DSIN in changing the system. As women are not in control of their contraceptive options to begin with, neither are they in control of ameliorating their personal and collective tragedies arising from their use of dangerous birth control methods. Nevertheless, the institutions of power are sensitive to the public actions and discourse that groups like DSIN engage in. Had DSIN not been involved in the process, many Dalkon Shield claimants might have received a smaller financial settlement.

The power of these activists resided in their successes in breaking the culture of silence, building a community, creating an open and public conflict with the official worldview, creating discourse with so many other social groups, and extending the larger issues of justice into the public domain.

6 Conclusions

The women who founded and led DSIN had no previous political experience and no organizing blueprints to follow. DSIN leaders reinvented the grass-roots organizing wheel and could have benefited from knowledge of other movements' successful tactics and strategies. Isolation and political naiveté exacerbate the problems faced by founders of social movements, yet many of them—like the women in this book— overcome their deficits in a remarkably short period of time. Although every social movement has a unique history and context that make it difficult to apply a generic set of rules for activism, change, and social justice, there are organizing guidelines that transcend context.

A MODEL CURRICULUM FOR EMPOWERMENT

The following discussion of tactics and strategies provides a generic template for any grass-roots group trying to organize into a collective with the means to inform, educate, and empower others within their community.

Statement of Purpose

As in any successful educational curriculum, a grass-roots group must develop a positively oriented organizational mission statement and an explicit set of goals based on an assessment of the needs of the identified community. The goals will contribute to articulating a working agenda for the group. The group must define, in concrete terms, what "justice" would entail if they could accomplish it. These goals will guide the energy and resource expenditures of the group. As the

group and the external circumstances surrounding the dynamics of
the issues evolve, these goals may be modified, added to, or dropped.

Division of Labor

It would be ideal for the leaders to negotiate a division of labor that
considers the various individual skills and talents of the group members. This allotment of tasks should be agreed upon in advance by
everyone. The division of labor would include persons or a small team
managing the following areas:

1. Generating written documents for distribution, including press
    statements
2. Recruiting membership and searching for funding
3. Organizing work crews and labor for mailing blitzes or tele-
    phone campaigns
4. Acting as ambassadors to establish rapport with other groups
    and allies
5. Offering telephone support and outreach to other persons in
    the target community

Personal Commitment

Founding members must be conscious of the numerous and often
chaotic demands that active involvement in a social cause will create.
There are never enough volunteers or resources, especially at the
beginning of any political campaign. Movement leaders can expect
to be physically and emotionally challenged by the intense demands
of breaking a culture of silence and publicly naming the problem they
advocate for. I strongly recommend that persons whose lives have
been characterized by chaos and emotional turmoil, and who themselves have been victimized in a tragic way, carefully evaluate the level
and the boundaries of their participation. They may need to do this
with the aid of a competent therapist, preferably one with an understanding of post-traumatic stress disorder.

Movement leaders who are part of a family group should also
negotiate limits of their participation with their significant others.
These people *will* be impacted, and they will be required to make
sacrifices that include the absence of the movement leader. Participation in a social movement disrupts personal lives, not only that of
the individual committed to the movement but also those of uncom-

mitted family members. Ignoring this aspect of movement leadership is inadvisable: Severe strain on or even the breakup of personal relationships may result from the intensive and all-consuming effort in which movement leaders will become involved.

Resources and Funding

From a practical standpoint, computers and telecommunications equipment are essential, even indispensable, to a group's ability to execute its agenda and disseminate its message effectively, particularly if national exposure is desired. The group members should decide to obtain as many of the following as possible:

Funds for incorporation fees at the state level, which enhances
the legitimacy of the organization
A word processor, preferably with desktop publishing and mail-
ing list management software, and a printer
A simple photocopier
A fax machine
A dedicated telephone line with call forwarding, call waiting, and
conference call features
A combination telephone and answering machine for that line

The prices of these items at discount stores are now substantially lower than they were in the late 1980s. Although grants from foundations generally do not cover capital equipment, the investment in most of these items is warranted. (If money is plentiful, it is certainly preferable to rent office space, acquire the items above, and hire at least one part-time staff person to assume the secretarial burdens.) The lack of a dedicated phone line, photocopier, and fax machine hindered DSIN's ability to be fully responsive. The great amount of time and energy required to use public copiers and fax machines was a significant burden on the few people conducting the group's business in the early days.

Other items that signal serious intent to potential supporters and group members include a checking account in the name of the organization and printed letterhead, preferably listing the names and titles of all leaders and a board of directors (where a board exists). It is certainly desirable for the group to obtain tax-exempt status. However, this process is more complex and lengthy than the process of incorporation, and the restrictions placed on organizations that receive this privilege should be carefully evaluated. It may be better as a long-term goal.

The careful development of financial resources is critical to long-term group survival and requires the energies of at least one person. There is an art and a science to both membership solicitation and grant acquisition, but they can be learned quickly with assistance and must be addressed from the earliest moments of a group's life.

Documents

Three types of written materials are indispensable to organizational promotion and growth: (1) a simple brochure describing the group, (2) a short document on the "history" of the problem or injustice, and (3) a periodic newsletter. The brochure can be a single piece of paper folded into thirds. The essential components must include the group's mission statement and goals, a listing of resource persons (with complete addresses and phone numbers), a list of written materials the group can provide (at minimal cost) on various topics, and a simple, tear-off membership application.

A short pamphlet on the history of the problem should be developed at the outset. It is critical to spend sufficient time developing this piece to ensure careful attention to detail and accuracy and to cite respected experts who are acknowledged prominently. All resource persons should also be listed, with complete addresses and telephone or fax numbers. This piece can be sent to every potential ally, funding sponsor, and press person; it will establish the group as a dependable and reliable source of information on the subject.

Producing a newsletter is essential to communication about the group to both internal and external constituencies. Contributed articles written from the perspective of the affected persons, in their own words, should be given highest priority. The language of the newsletter should be nontechnical and nonacademic, evoking the greatest prospect of collective identification. Every issue of the newsletter should contain a list of resources and resource persons on the various aspects of the case. At least one article should be a summary of the group's activities; it could be sent to other allied groups, who may then reprint it in their own newsletters or publications. In any event, the newsletter should be mailed free of charge to all organizations perceived as allies.

It is also desirable to develop a list of written materials, by title, on various topics of interest to the population, and to make it widely available at some nominal price. These items might include a pamphlet on the history of the case, any books that may have been written on the subject, back issues of the group's newsletters, and a series of fact sheets that deal with different aspects in the case.

Developing Allies

The single most important activity of an embryonic organization is the cultivation and maintenance of positive, constructive internal and external relationships. This is more important than doctrine and ideology. The "old boys' network" is a testimony to the strength of carefully constructed relationships. People who may seem peripheral to a group at one moment may later become crucial allies. Every external contact person or group must be added to the permanent mailing list and must receive copies of all newsletters or general publications, whether they ask for them or not! The future engagement of allies will be facilitated by keeping all potential allies informed of the group's business.

Early brainstorming sessions should address how to link a seemingly single issue to larger issues of social justice and how to devise a means for establishing and maintaining communications with representatives of sympathetic existing organizations that advocate reform on related issues. There should be no presumption concerning "natural" allies, nor should there be discouragement about low numbers of external supporters for the new cause. A sad trend in our era is shrinking financial resources for countless numbers of worthy causes involving human welfare, and the competition for scarce resources is keen.

An important phase for the group will be when it makes decisions about political alliances; leaders must carefully assess groups that do extend some type of outreach to them. The subtleties of external group legitimacy and agendas must be evaluated thoroughly and astutely. It is also important to distinguish among *friends*, *allies*, and *coalitions*. The differing levels of relationships with other groups require that the impact of joint efforts on the group's identity be deliberately assessed.

Membership

A constant challenge is how to engage other members of the target community in the cause and the organization. An elaborate, predetermined doctrine may inhibit the empowerment of newcomers. All written materials from the organization should be able to speak to a person who is totally uninformed about the issue. These materials must be constantly revised as the group gains more experience and builds its own information base, but new members will need introductory information similar to that which the group first developed to define itself. As each new aspect of the case is faced and dealt with, a series of fact sheets, or position papers, should be drafted and eventually added to the list of publications; these fact sheets will reduce the time required to update the uninformed. Absorbing information is also an important step in the empowerment of newcomers.

Pivotal Events

An embryonic group must plan and execute a pivotal first event, one that effects the public naming of the problem and presents potential remedies. Other events of affirmation must continue to be held. There are specific windows of opportunity that will attract press coverage, if that is desired. Tracking news through the *Wall Street Journal* or the *New York Times* will aid in making decisions about the best timing for public events. It is also possible to create news by staging a proactive event, for example, a ceremony inducting persons or companies into a "Hall of Shame." Specific objectives for each event should be established to ensure the desired effect of the event. Pictorial symbols and logos are extremely useful, both for purposes of identification among the community and for the media.

In the case of a widely dispersed membership, the availability of electronic methods such as videoconferencing should be considered a partial remedy to the costs of travel and the problem of reaching large numbers of the target community. Financial considerations may limit what can be accomplished in that regard, but this medium *must* become more useful in building collectives.

Assessment

Every internal and external action of a new group has a lesson, or learning opportunity. In order for a group to keep to its task, and to maintain positive and productive relationships while moving toward organization goals, it must constantly evaluate and reflect upon both internal and external experiences. By this means mistakes are transmuted to opportunities for improvement. There should be conscious, deliberate dialogue among the members on this point.

Evaluation of the group's functioning should be ongoing and

brutally honest. In a small and geographically intact working group, it is easier to maintain this type of dialogue. DSIN leaders participating in public events spent hours, if not days, assessing strong and weak points in the execution of public events. At an early stage of a grassroots social movement, the reviewing of past events should be built into planning for the future. Everything is a building block and nothing should be defined as a failure; the inevitable mistakes should be framed as opportunities for the group to grow stronger.

A CLEARINGHOUSE FOR EMPOWERMENT

Tudiver (1986) gives an overview of the phenomenal achievements of women's health action groups and the links among various groups around the world, all of which fight abuses of the pharmaceutical industry and medical violence against women. She also points out the considerable energy and commitment of women to get difficult jobs done. "That's nothing new; it's the elements out of which we've always made history" (p. 210). For Tudiver, the key to success in achieving reform is the collaboration of women consumers; health professionals; sympathetic, non-industry-sponsored researchers; and constituencies from the environmental, consumer, and international development movements. The common goal must be the rational use of pharmaceuticals on a worldwide scale.

The women's health movement has had an important effect on health care. From its position outside the system, the women's health movement was able to pressure the system to respond. The original goals of women-centered, women-controlled health care are still vital today. The need to emphasize wellness, preventive health care, and gaining higher social status for women in general is perhaps even more pressing than it was in the 1970s, as we witness the spiraling costs of health care and what is called the backlash against women's achievements in the last 20 years (Faludi, 1991). However, the power and influence of women in the medical arena would be greater if these diverse groups were more closely aligned. There are already models or solutions to the abuses of medicine, but better mechanisms for engaging and harnessing the energies of the masses of women are urgently needed.

I recommend the creation of an entity to be a *clearinghouse of empowerment* for all women's health groups and organizations. The Citizens Clearinghouse on Hazardous Waste (CCHW), headed by Lois

Gibbs, is an excellent prototype. CCHW aids in the creation of grass-roots groups all over the United States and offers technical assistance to would-be organizers, precisely for empowerment. It provides experts, consulting advice, and a plethora of publications on environmental justice to help neophyte organizers establish themselves in their region. CCHW also publishes a newsletter that reports all those activities, and it sponsors an annual meeting featuring a variety of workshops on empowerment. To my knowledge and from my experience, a similar mechanism for facilitating empowerment for activism does not exist in the women's health movement. Both the National Women's Health Network (NWHN) and the Boston Women's Health Book Collective (BWHBC) provide important information on health issues, and the enormous success of BWHBC's book *Our Bodies, Ourselves* has addressed the empowerment of women; but these organizations have not developed mechanisms that can empower large numbers of women in working groups at the grass-roots level. Their advocacy is currently limited, on behalf of "women," to the priorities of their boards and staff members. The participation of many more women could be increased by incorporating the passionate energies of survivors of medical abuse and by capitalizing on the enthusiasm of women who do reach out to the existing organizations.

This type of organizational structure would also allow for a more coordinated response to new threats of medical abuse and to legislative initiatives involving women's health care reform, which often require applying pressure to Congress. Ralph Nader and his organizations have achieved a large degree of success fighting corporate-sponsored tort reform. Consumer and victim groups are kept informed of developments on pending legislation and are even invited to attend national press conferences, which Nader organizes at sensitive political moments. He brings together many single-issue organizations and harnesses their energy toward a common goal. This dynamic could be—*must* be—developed in order to bring greater political pressure to bear on and more responsive legislative action on issues of women's health care reform.

Bookman and Morgen (1988) chronicle the grass-roots accomplishments of women in instituting reform and suggest that a combination of grass-roots and electoral strategies may achieve even greater social change:

> Whether the social-change strategy is electoral or grassroots, women are organizing in ways that challenge both prevailing conceptions of state

responsibility and the traditional, male preserves that have excluded women from the political process. (p. 320)

THE POWER OF THE PURSE

In addition to legislative lobbying and being elected to political office, women can and must go directly to the political economic powers, that is, corporate America. The controlling elites at the top of the capitalist pyramid are more vulnerable than is acknowledged or appreciated by the general public. Women purchase most pharmaceutical products, not only for themselves but for the entire household. Two examples from 1989 alone demonstrate this untapped potential of activist groups. The first example was the stranglehold of anti-choice groups on the pharmaceutical industry with regard to the importation of RU-486 into the United States (Fraser, 1988). The second example involves the AIDS activists in the group Act-Up, who are widely credited with effecting enormous changes in the availability and distribution of the drug AZT by using radical guerrilla tactics aimed at the pharmaceutical industry; for example, members chained themselves inside the New York Stock Exchange, and they have also staged aggressive protest actions outside governmental health agencies.

The political strategies and tactics for bringing direct pressures to bear on economic elites are numerous. Such possibilities were not tapped in the Dalkon Shield case. Perhaps a well-crafted and well-timed threat of a product boycott could have led to direct negotiations with women or indirect repercussions and benefits. DSIN leaders thrashed through many plans for damaging the image of other Robins products. One DSIN leader even made a covert visit to Robins's Richmond headquarters in order to glean valuable information for planning purposes. Also, several plans to demonstrate directly in front of Robins's corporate headquarters, using guerrilla-theater tactics, were not acted upon. Additionally, Dalkon Shield women could all have bought at least one share of A. H. Robins stock and then insinuated themselves into the annual shareholders' meetings and business. At the very least, they would have received shareholder information, which would have aided in planning counterstrategies.

Grass-roots strategies can be developed to confront and challenge economic elites directly. The ideals of democracy and human rights are more evident among many grass-roots and public interest organizations such as DSIN than in the actions of many governmental officials, who promote the agendas of the special-interest groups that finance their campaigns.

WOMEN AND SOCIAL MOVEMENTS

Women are at the center of movements for change, including the peace and justice, antinuclear, civil rights, and environmental movements. Academic and societal debate continues about whether or not women have superior qualities that men should aspire to in order to make political life more humane, fair, and just (Miller, 1986). The media portrayed the 1992 elections in the United States as "The Year of the Woman in Politics." As noted in other studies of women's movements (Blumberg & West, 1989) and confirmed in this book, women's motivations for becoming politically engaged often stem from aspects of gender socialization, specifically their maternal instincts to be passionate about the welfare of others—the ethic of care. The feeling that no one else is "out there" fighting for such issues contributes to the urgency to get involved.

Political inexperience and naiveté put many women at an initial disadvantage when it comes to taking the political action demanded by circumstances such as those surrounding the Dalkon Shield case. However, the considerable personal resources and skills in relationship building, which are generally attributed to women, allowed them to "catch up" and to begin acting quickly in a politically astute fashion. If we accept the premise that women are socialized to excel at the cultivation and maintenance of relationships or affiliations (Gilligan, 1982), then we must also see women as an asset to any political action group's development and success. The interpersonal skills required for the development and maintenance of relationships will enhance any group's potential for success. The clues and cues inherent in social relations that women pay close attention to can be used to advantage in conducting political action and planning an action agenda.

The Dalkon Shield women described in this book learned, through painful experience, how to deal with confrontation and adversarial relations. At least for most of these women, this skill was largely lacking from their early life experiences. Since their backgrounds and socialization did emphasize nurturing relationships, it was difficult for them to engage in adversarial relations without experiencing emotional pain. The single most important lesson we learned from experience, however, was not to waste time and limited energy fighting noncooperating groups or groups with incompatible agendas.

Energy and resources should be expended on accomplishing a group's stated goals, not on tearing down or trashing someone else's actions. The feminist literature decries the pheonomenon called *trashing*, as if women should not be vulnerable to using tactics that defame the character of their opponents. The behavior of men toward their opponents in political campaigns certainly dramatizes the ubiquity of the tendency to use defamation of character in political battlegrounds. Although obliteration of this behavior is a noble goal that both men and women should strive to achieve, it is important for women to expect trashing to occur and not to be paralyzed or distracted from their goals upon learning that others may be working against them. Fragmentation within a social movement can and should be viewed as a healthy and productive development if intragroup tensions have rendered a group stagnant or ineffective in achieving its goals. In spite of ethical or philosophical differences that may preclude unity among the various splinter groups that often arise, I continue to believe that every group contributes something beneficial to the community and to the overall resolution of the issue. Destroying the work of others will only jeopardize a group's own effectiveness, identity, and legitimacy, as well as benefit the common enemy.

The social and peer pressure on women not to rise above the group (of other women) also inhibits them from acting with more authority and trusting their own judgments to take bold stands and exhibit incisive leadership. We must learn to support women who do rise above the group. This is the double-edged sword: We must be in relationships with others and yet be able to act boldly and courageously although our actions may be contrary to the wishes of the group—and to do so without creating paralyzing anxiety.

The women described in this book struggled with issues that characterize men's political behavior. They developed hierarchies of power and became enmeshed in power and control issues. Ruzek's (1978) analysis of the women's health movement and studies of the women's political movement in the 1960s and 1970s (Carden, 1974; Davis, 1991; Freeman, 1975) also refer to this phenomenon, even among groups whose organizing principles may have been overtly expressed as egalitarian. Therefore, I conclude that gender is a necessary but insufficient variable to explain the political actions and strategies of women. Women are susceptible to the same personal dynamics of leadership that characterize men's politics.

Politics includes any attempt to change the social and economic institutions that embody the basic power relations in society (Bookman & Morgen, 1988). Social protest movements are a particular form of politics. The difference between the protest movements and politics is in the strategies used as vehicles to power. Social protesters conduct their politics outside the formal institutions of power, which generally exclude them from direct participation in matters vital to their welfare. Persons engaged in social movements impose themselves into a process that has marginalized or excluded them.

Social protest movements, like electoral politics, involve the engagement of energy and resources in the public forum. They create and sustain a public discourse among different constituencies, representing and furthering the needs, rights, and interests of an oppressed group. All groups participating in the public forum aim to have some impact on or effect change in the formal legislative and legal institutions of power—and this is a political undertaking.

Involvement in political action groups transforms women. It creates changes in political consciousness, in women's relations with other women and with men, and in the ways women perceive their relationship to the structures of economic and political power (Bookman & Morgen, 1988). "These changes transcend the categories of winning and losing and place women unquestionably at a critical juncture in contemporary politics" (Bookman & Morgen, p. 315).

DSIN leaders never expected to win. They interrupted the official worldview, however, to give voice to the victims of injustice. They began acting without knowing the complexity of the issues and the special interests that underlay the case; and when they became aware of this, it intensified their determination and turned them into passionate, committed warriors. Attaining a level of experience with and competence in politics may lead some DSIN activists into more public arenas that they might not otherwise have imagined entering. These women survived a living hell and transformed it into a vision of a better world.

Epilogue

Contraceptive technology is a quality-of-life issue. It is not therapy for pathology, yet controlling women's fertility has moved into the disease model of medicine. High-tech birth control methods remove women's reproductive control and connect women patients on a regular basis to the medical care system. When the focus of a medical value system is technology, the emphasis is not on empowering individuals but on creating dependence and imposing social control through medicine (Scully, 1980, in press). Birth control has become a commodity of great value to the interests of physicians, pharmaceutical companies, family planning and population control agencies, and the government (Petchesky, 1984).

HIGH-TECH CONTRACEPTION

That combination of elites looks at the lessons of the Dalkon Shield case through a lens that is opposed to the interests of the injured women. A rash of articles in 1990 lamented the lag of "modern" contraceptives (hormonal implants, injectables, and copper-bearing IUDs) in the United States relative to most other countries in the developing world (Bacon, 1990; Lichtenstein, 1990; Roberts, 1990). The fear of liability is cited as the major impediment to their more widespread distribution among U.S. women. These articles do not address the long-term health implications or demonstrate concern for the effects of these products on women's bodies.

The pharmaceutical industry is poised to profit handsomely from a more extensive use of high tech birth control methods in the United States. Oral and injectable contraceptives are among the most lucrative of *all* pharmaceuticals (Sun, 1982). Two types were recently approved by the FDA. In 1991 Norplant, the 5-year subdermal hormonal implant, was approved. In October 1992, the Upjohn Corporation finally won its long battle for the approval for Depo Provera, the hormonal injectable. The dangers of Depo Provera and Norplant have been known and debated for more than 15 years (Hardon & Achthoven, 1990; "Health Department Backs Off . . . ," 1992; Joseph, 1992; Neil, 1992; Scully, 1980, in press). Yet a member of the Population Crisis Committee, in a television interview, called the approval of Depo Provera a victory for U.S. women, who now can have the same choices as women in Bangladesh.

Family-planning agency materials that address contraceptive risk factors always focus on comparing mortality (death) rates of women using the specific birth control method to mortality rates connected to pregnancy and birthing, while trivializing or even ignoring morbidity (illness) rates. This focus obscures the fact that very real dangers of serious iatrogenesis exist. A recent research report on IUDs and pelvic inflammatory disease (PID), sponsored by the World Health Organization, illustrates how this trivialization occurs. According to Farley, Rosenberg, Rowe, Chen, and Meirik (1992), some 84 million women around the world were using IUDs in 1987. By applying the PID rates cited among the Farley study's subjects to this total number of worldwide IUD users, almost 300,000 women could be expected to develop detectable PID. However, glaring omissions in the study have undoubtedly underestimated the extent of the total adverse outcomes: The study excluded women in known high-risk categories and all cases of device removal for reasons other than PID. Therefore, information is not available on such injuries as ectopic pregnancy, septic abortions, and so forth. The extent of the injuries that were diagnosed is not recorded, which means there is no information about women who required surgery, who were rendered infertile, or who died. The number of women who were lost to follow-up is not included in the report.

These study data indicate geographical differences, with African women suffering the highest rates of PID. "Low-tech" women using high-tech contraception in developing countries or urban ghettos must be particularly vulnerable, since clinical follow-up, skilled staff, and expensive antibiotics are not available. The added problem of poor means of communication for notification about problems in such countries, dramatically demonstrated in the Dalkon Shield case (discussed in Chapter 2), should make high-tech contraception unacceptable in these areas.

With access to safe, legal abortion again threatened in the United States in the 1980s and 1990s, leaders of the feminist movement have opted to join the power elites in proclaiming these new birth control products as a victory for choice. On two other occasions in this century, feminists helped men to gain a greater degree of control over women's reproductive lives. Margaret Sanger, the founder of the modern birth control movement, allied herself with physicians and eugenicists in order to gain legitimacy for her work (Gordon, 1977). In the 1970s, feminists were slow to react to the sterilization abuse experienced by women of color because of the needed alliance of population control agencies in the fight for abortion rights (Ruzek, 1978).

In the 1990s, a third such occasion arose, this time involving the drug RU-486. Eleanor Smeal, president of the Feminist Majority Foundation, has led the campaign for the introduction of RU-486 into the United States by calling on all college students, scientists, and academicians to lobby on behalf of this abortifacient. These endorsements are extremely useful to the pharmaceutical industry. Their activities have included staging high-profile press conferences with scientists at Roussel Uclaf, the pharmaceutical firm that developed RU-486. Smeal's written literature praises the drug repeatedly as a "safe and simple" method of fertility control. It is doubtful that Roussel Uclef could make the same claims without fearing product-liability litigation. The rhetoric of an April 1990 fundraising letter signed by Smeal is reminiscent of the Dalkon Shield advertising literature: "We cannot allow opponents of women's rights to hold hostage medical technology *that will improve the lives of millions of women* in the United States and around the world" (emphasis added).

When Raymond, Klein, and Dumble (1991) issued a report questioning the long-term safety issues related to RU-486, Smeal resorted to trashing Raymond (a former nun and founder of Catholics for a Free Choice) in a *Science* interview by suggesting that she "has links to organizations that have been critical of abortion in general" (Hoffman, 1991, p. 199). This personal attack on a prominent pro-choice activist has the effect of ignoring the necessary attention to safety concerns and distracting feminists from important issues related to this potent drug. A more constructive approach to this timely and necessary debate, based on the scientifically relevant arguments, surfaced in the National Women's Health Network *Network News*, where both sides of the safety question were presented (Callum, 1992; Klein et al., 1992).

RECOMMENDATIONS ON SAFETY ISSUES

To allow healthy women to risk iatrogenic illness from high-tech contraceptives is unconscionable. The notion that women in the developing world have better contraceptives obscures the fact that there is a substantial misuse of potent drugs, a lack of regulation, and unacceptable conduct associated with clinical trials outside the United States (Ehrenreich et al., 1979; Hartmann, 1987; "Health Department Backs Off . . . ," 1992; Joseph, 1992; Raymond et al., 1991; Tudiver, 1986). Diethylstilbestrol (DES) is still being given to women in developing countries for inappropriate indications (Hoen, 1990). Norplant, Depo Provera, and many other products require a good health care infrastructure, which simply does not exist in many developing countries, particularly in rural areas.

Allowing the proliferation of these products because scientific evidence is inconclusive amounts to an abuse of power and privilege, as well as a continuing pattern of exploitation and medical violence against women. Furthermore, corporate and medical interests control and manage the negative information in a deliberate way. Adverse outcomes are still ignored or trivialized. Breakthrough bleeding, headaches, nausea, and weight gain experienced by birth control pill users are referred to as "nuisance" side effects ("Experts debate . . . ," 1992), yet studies show that 50% to 60% of American women discontinue their use of pills due to these outcomes. Even the use of the term "*side*" *effects* diminishes the importance of these adverse outcomes relative to the medical intent of avoiding pregnancy.

The secrecy surrounding the Dalkon Shield Claimants Trust, which has not released specific data related to the global nature and extent of injuries, continues to exacerbate the problems that Dalkon Shield women have in securing high financial awards and in managing the diseases that so many of them have. Access to that database would generate a wealth of vital information about the side effects of IUDs, as well as the extensive medical mismanagement involved in contraception.

Men, children, and extended families were also adversely affected by the women's physical injuries. The voices of these people are entirely submerged. An accounting of their stories would clarify the devastating effects that this contraceptive had, not only on women's bodies but also on the lives of entire family groups. Some men also suffered a vicarious type of infertility in cases in which women's reproductive organs were completely destroyed by the damage from the Shield. The statement by Russell Stone about his missed opportunity for fatherhood eloquently expresses a man's pain. (See Appendix C.) Parents of injured women dealt with the pain of knowing they would never become grandparents. Some men were widowed. No one has ever chronicled the effects of these traumas on relationships.

It is vital for women to continue to challenge the arrogance of the power elites about these matters. Additionally, I propose four ways to promote greater accountability on the issue of health and welfare related to contraceptives.

1. The executives of pharmaceutical companies and population control agencies who develop and distribute products must be made personally accountable to the public. Named individuals, not faceless corporations, should be associated with all safety claims. There must be legislation to create a workable system of criminal indictments and convictions against persons who deceive or lie to the public. Today civil penalties are the only deterrent; yet organized medicine and the pharmaceutical industry have responded to the Dalkon Shield case by ensuring a reduction of their financial liabilities.

   Furthermore, the substantial economic costs of contraceptive iatrogenesis should be calculated and acknowledged. The losses of income and earning potential, as well as the devastating effect of a woman's illness on the family unit, are considerable. No reduction in financial liabilities can be tolerated. The existing tort system must be maintained in the absence of a better alternative. Potential financial penalties do apply some degree of pressure to the industry.

2. It is essential to establish a national registry system for birth control and other pharmaceutical products. If it is possible to develop a computerized system for registering car parts and recalling defective tires, we can offer women greater guarantees against harm through a program of notification and corrective action for the drugs they ingest and devices they use. The registry must be maintained by a consumer advocacy mechanism that is totally independent of pharmaceutical and corporate interests. This system would provide a huge database that could also be used to construct the proper and necessary studies related to long-term use, improve the problem of inadequate follow-up, and allow for early warnings that would diminish iatrogenesis, infertility, and death. This system would actually even benefit the pharmaceutical industry by limiting its jeopardy.

3. The FDA is a weak and ineffectual agency and must be overhauled,

through congressional action, so that it has greater authority to evaluate new drugs and medical devices. Regarding experimental study protocols on new drugs, Haire (1984) notes that the FDA routinely accepts the manufacturer's data on drug safety at face value. Data accepted by the FDA may be prepared by researchers who are in the employ of the drug's manufacturer.

In Haire's opinion, things are worse now than they were in 1984. "The FDA does not even have a specific requirement of the company to provide the informed consent form offered to the subject in an experiemental study," she observes (personal communication, November 6, 1992). For 20 years, Haire has fought hard for patient package inserts for prescription medications, which are still not mandatory. She fights an uphill battle for fuller disclosure to consumers. She continues to insist that the inserts include a statement about the lack of information on long-term effects of new drugs.

The FDA must strengthen its standards on drugs and devices sold for quality-of-life uses (as opposed to cures for diseases). Until that happens, the FDA must be held liable, in the same manner as the pharmaceutical companies, for negligence in protecting the public health. Its abominable record of many failures should serve as the basis for naming the agency as a co-defendant in product-liability litigation.

4. A greater share of resources must be applied to research and development on other methods and mechanisms of birth control. This would include male methods, barrier methods, and other novel approaches, such as immunocontraception. The urgent need to limit or eradicate the spread of sexually transmitted diseases should be perceived as an additional incentive to improve barrier methods. The lack of interest in, commitment to, and funding for these approaches can be correlated to low profits and the continuing sexism that causes a reticence to experiment on men's bodies. From a strictly economic viewpoint, the low costs associated with these methods should be as attractive to the public sector as they are unattractive to the private sector.

GLOBAL POPULATION PRESSURES

The world's population pressures cannot be ignored or minimized. Population control experts, however, opt for a narrow focus on the total control of women's fertility to solve population dilemmas. David

Eschenbach (1992), a leading gynecologist who researches IUDs and PID, recently challenged his professional colleagues to own up to the fact that IUDs cause PID and that women should not have to pay the price of losing their fertility because of them. Other controversies involving population growth include issues such as land ownership and redistribution, employment, education, and the status of women generally (Hartmann, 1987). To Hartmann, population control has become a substitute for social justice.

It would be very profitable for the pharmaceutical industry to gain total control of women's hormones. It is possible to manage each woman's entire hormonal function with synthetic chemicals. The normal menstrual cycle, increasingly framed as a nuisance, can be and often is managed by prescribing birth control pills, even when there is no need for contraception. Advertisements in medical literature and the popular press recommend permanent estrogen replacement therapy for *all* menopausal women. High-tech infertility treatments manipulate the menstrual cycle in order for a woman to achieve a pregnancy. This aggressive, invasive approach to managing the entire lifetime functioning of women's reproductive systems is increasingly attractive to many, in spite of the inconclusive, contradictory, and often nonexistent evidence about the effects of these chemicals on women's bodies.

Population demography must not look only at birth and death rates. It is a grave failing to omit, or to ignore, the sickness that precedes death from defective and dangerous contraception. More attention needs to be focused on the varying social and cultural settings in which women find themselves. The International Group on Women and Pharmaceuticals is developing guidelines on the distribution and use of high-tech contraceptives, which include stringent monitoring and supervision of the programs that dispense them. Assessments of contraceptive technology must not make women expendable in the grander scheme of things.

Appendix A
Interview with Fran Cleary

Karen Hicks (KH): Why were you so alone in Richmond? Other Dalkon Shield women never got in touch with you, especially with all the press coverage you did in Richmond, but women there never contacted you.

Fran Cleary (FC): I know, I think about that all the time. In Richmond, the Robins company is so big, a gigantic company, and people are afraid, afraid to identify themselves and maybe losing their case or getting hurt professionally. One woman I did talk to was just petrified; she didn't want anyone at her work to know anything—that she had anything to do with DSIN—because she was afraid if they found out, her job would be in jeopardy; they would think she was creating a lot of problems, and I think problems mainly for the community, as opposed to other people who lived in different cities, this wouldn't be a problem if they spoke out. The fact that Robins has the McGuire, Woods, and Battle law firm representing them, and that is a very *powerful* and large law firm, or at least it was; it still is but not as much as when they blew it with the Robins case; they also have a lot of power, and then you're talking about Judge Merhige supporting them— he has a lot of power; so you add all these things up, and I think women didn't want to get involved in that.

KH: How come you got involved in our group (DSIN)?

FC: I guess for one thing, I'm not the average person, in the sense that those kinds of things don't frighten me. I'm a homemaker, I haven't had a job for years. My husband's job is such that it wouldn't affect his job. I had no fears along those lines. I also had a lot of bitterness about the whole thing. Part of that was not related to my physical problems. It was also related to the fact that my former father-in-law, who had been the vice-president of Robins, had lied to me. That really fueled my fire.

KH: How did you find out that your former father-in-law played this role at Robins?

FC: How I found out about it is directly related to you and what you did for me, really, because I'm glad I found out about it. You, the DSIN, sent a group of women to the records facility to get names, to get a following, or a group of people together. Fortunately for me, my name was one of the names you found, and I know you only found a small percentage, I mean a pittance of the numbers. My name was one of them. I got a letter in the mail telling me about your organization, and that you were having a rally here in July [1987]. Well, at the time of the mailing, we were getting ready to go out of town and I didn't have time to do anything about it and couldn't go to the rally.

When I got back, I saw this mail sitting on my desk and I thought, well, I'll join this organization. I'd like to learn more about it. So I sent you the membership fee, and in return, you sent me a book called *Nightmare*, and when I read the book, I found out that my former father-in-law had written a memo that had blown this whole thing wide open when it was found by the courts in Minnesota, when they came to the Robins Company and found these documents. He had written it in 1970 and it stated that there might be a problem with wicking.

It was *after* that time that he was very adamant about me having the Shield put in and really convinced me it was safe and wonderful. . . . I can remember specific questions that my ex-husband and I asked him about it; he answered the questions in lies, and he had already written this memo to the company saying this wicking problem needed to be investigated. That was bad enough and I couldn't really believe it, and I called you and we discussed it and you said there's another book written by Morton Mintz and maybe I should check that. So you gave me Morton's phone number and I called him, discussed it with him, he told me, yes, that was the correct date, and he would send me a copy of his book, and he did and he gave me the phone number of Bradley Post, and that I should call Post, and I did, and I had a nice discussion with him about it, and he explained in great detail how he had found the memo and everything else, and this . . . I mean, it really blew my mind. I was very traumatized by this for months . . . I mean I didn't sleep well, I kept thinking about it constantly, and I still do.

My father-in-law is deceased, so I can't ask him why he did this . . . I can't get the answers I'd like to have about it. I remember one occasion, my mother-in-law—his wife—said to me once about tampons that I shouldn't be wearing them in the bathtub because the water could wick up—she used the word, *wick*—could wick up the tampon string and cause infections . . . when she told me that, in his presence, he just became totally livid. This was probably about two years after [my injury]. He just like, went screaming at her "You don't know what you're talking about—shut your mouth!!!" Where did she hear it? He must have mentioned something to her about it . . . probably not the Shield . . . anyway, he knew. All that time, he knew. That just proved to me that he knew, and then he didn't tell me. When we asked questions that he could have answered, he didn't.

I have an aunt who came to visit us over the holidays this year, and she used to work for the Robins company. She now lives in Texas and hasn't worked there [at Robins] for a long time. She knew my father-in-law when she worked for them, and she said, "Well, you know what it is . . . that company was so different than your average company, and unless you work there, you can't understand this." But she said that loyalties were so strong at that company because the Robins family made a big point, making a big thing, of taking care of their employees, and they did it very well. She said when you work for them, it was a family, and you wouldn't do anything to harm your family. And she said that was what he was doing, and I think she's right. His loyalties were greater to them than to his own family. And I think that's probably what it amounts to; not to mention the fact that there was a lot financially to gain, and he was a businessman. I think the combination of those two things. . . .

And I know I've told you this before but I'll repeat this to you is the fact that he died of a brain tumor and he'd been sick for quite a while. My ex-husband and I used to come to Richmond (we lived in another city at that time) while he was ill and take care of him and help his wife with the care because he was pretty bad. When he was in the hospital the last time, he had meningitis and he was very ill and needed a lot of extra care, so we came and relieved his wife, told her to go home, that we would take care of him. My ex-husband went to get coffee and I was there, mopping his brow and taking care of him next to his bed, and he grabbed my hand and squeezed it, wouldn't let go, and he kept saying over and over again, "I'm sorry, I'm sorry, I'm sorry." He was so ill, he was dying of a brain tumor, and I did not know what he was talking about at the time. I did not understand. I thought this was pretty weird. Then, my former husband came back into the room and said "What's the matter?" and I said I didn't know, he just kept telling me he was sorry. Then he let go and went to sleep, and we left the room, and the next time anybody saw him, which was the nurse, he was dead. And I think he was apologizing to me for what had happened to me. . . .

It didn't dawn on me until *after* I found out about this from read-ing the book, in August 1987, that's when I joined your organization, that's when you sent me the book, that's when I found out. I woke up one night . . . I mean, I couldn't sleep, thinking about this all the time. Then I woke up one night and I remembered that incident, and I went, "Oh, my God, this is why he was doing this! 'Cause he knew all the time! All that for his success, and he felt guilty about it . . . he felt guilty all the time he was doing it apparently. And that was in 1974, and very shortly after he died was when it was taken off the market.

KH: Is it very important for you to continue getting information?

FC: Yes, I still have questions I'd love to have answers to. Before I knew all this, I wasn't traumatized because I didn't realize that this was the case. I just thought, well, I've been injured by something, I wasn't even certain.

KH: What is the effect on you now, looking back just since 1987, having this information to put these pieces together? What does it mean to you?

FC: For one thing, finding out that, coupled with the knowledge I gained by getting involved with you and going to the court situa-tion, learning more about the whole situation, has definitely soured my attitude toward justice in this country. It's changed my attitude toward businesses and the way people operate; trusting people and a lot of things like that.

It soured me, and I'm bitter about it, and I've become more bit-ter about a lot of things as a consequence, and that's not good but that's the way it is. The fact that I was lied to for so many years by someone I loved, and who loved me, and that money and success meant more than the truth, and after I found this out, I saw it again and again in the courts, when the Robins company was continually trying to use the women who were injured and turned around and made them look like the guilty parties, when all along they knew they were the guilty parties, and they continued to do that all along, and they're still doing it right up to this day.

I don't think Robins Sr. or Jr. have ever admitted that they made a mistake, even when they were asked to by the court, they still haven't done it. Even Merhige asked E. Claiborne, Jr., to say he was sorry and he basically wouldn't do it. And that kind of thing has made me very bitter about the whole thing, and I'm still bitter. I think the attitude is . . . well, when you start to lie, when you state a lie, it becomes reality in your mind. You have to make that become reality in order to live with yourself, and that's what they were doing.

And I think that's what happened with my father-in-law in a sense. He was trying to believe that there was nothing wrong with this product. He wanted to believe that very much. I think I'm more bitter with my personal experience, knowing that my father-in-law lied to me, than the average person would be having the same injuries that I have had.

When my former father-in-law was describing the virtues of the Dalkon Shield to me, he was totally obsessed with it. When we would go to visit, he would pull out his little briefcase with all this s— in it, he would show his clients. He was the vice-president for international marketing of the Dalkon Shield. He went to India and sold millions of the things . . . he went to lots of other countries, and his thrust was to get these things into poor people who came into the clinics, to control the population explosion. Well, anyway, he took this thing out and started playing with it, showing us how it was inserted . . . he had a false vagina and a false uterus, a little stick and look how it went in so easy, and just pull it out, which absolutely didn't work that way. So I would sit, I was trying to decide whether to use it or not.

I have a degree in biology and I wasn't just going to do whatever somebody told me. That's what makes it harder on me, because we had so many questions. And one of the questions I asked him was how long it had been tested. I asked him that question before I ever had it inserted. His answer was this . . . and it was an out and out *lie*, because here's the answer . . . "Well, you know that any drug (well, maybe he just twisted it around but he insinuated that this was a drug) has to be approved by the FDA and it takes 17 years of testing before they'll approve it." That was his answer. So, I assumed from that answer that that meant the Dalkon Shield had been tested all this time. So I said what are the statistics on pregnancy rates and things. And he said, "I'll tell you what I'm going to do . . . I'm going to give you a book about it so you can read all about it for yourself" (not to mention that I had asked him lots of other questions that he had answered, such as what are the side effects, are there any problems?). He said "Very few, no problems, the only problem is that it can perforate the uterus, that's the biggest problem. So you have to have a physician who is sure what he's doing, so I'm going to make arrangements for you to have yours put in by Dr. X, because he's already inserted 500 of them, and he knows what he's doing, because he's a consultant for the Robins Company. I'm going to call and make a personal appointment for you." Which he did.

And he gave me this book written by Hugh Davis. It was a very scientific-looking book. It looked very official. It was published by a reputable company, and I read it and it looked fine. The pregnancy rate was 1%. I gave the book to a friend of mine who was in medical school, and I called him to get the book back, because I really wanted that book, but he didn't have it anymore. I was very disappointed about that, because I would like to have my hands on that book. And he was clever about it. It's probably the answer he would give to a doctor who asked him any question. It immediately implies that it was a well-tested device, and it wasn't. And I blame the FDA in a large part for this happening. It should have never gotten on the market. But that's a whole other story.

As Morton Mintz said, these people were church-going citizens . . . my father-in-law was big in the church, big-time church goer, his father was a minister, and yet, he did this. He saw me dying in the hospital . . . he saw me lying in the bed with every kind of tube they make in me. That's why I am so curious now about what he did do. I told Morton Mintz that he must have written a memo to someone about this situation and urged them to do further testing, after my hospitalization, and it's possible that he did, but they destroyed all those documents, and now nobody will ever know that. I've got a lot of questions, and there are a lot of people I would like to talk to, but I don't want to keep dragging it out because I'm not going to change anything by having certain answers.

For instance, I haven't even talked to my ex-husband about this, and in a way, you know, he suffered a lot, having to go through all this. And if he knew that his father was responsible, it would be hard on him. I don't know if it would help him any, and I don't want to get back and get involved in that relationship again, anyway. I think it will really help if I just don't get too carried away . . . keep it in perspective because I was getting very carried away when I first found out about it. I was very upset and traumatized for months and I've gotten over that now, and I think the best thing for me to do is just try to keep it in perspective.

Appendix B
Chronology of the DSIN

Date	Court Events	DSIN Events
8/85	Robins is granted Chapter 11 status at court	
4/86	Court receives 332,000 Dalkon Shield claims	
1/87		1st newsletter published
2/87	American Home Products (AHP) makes offer to buy Robins, with $1.75 billion for Dalkon Shield Claims	
3/87	AHP withdraws offer	2nd newsletter published
4/87	Robins submits its own reorganization plan, with $1.75 billion for Dalkon Shield claims	
5/87		3rd newsletter published, Richmond rally plans, including 1st Richmond trip
6/87		Richmond rally preparations, including 3 Richmond trips
7/87	Robins and Rorer announce merger agreement, with $1.75 billion for Dalkon Shield claims	Richmond rally: protest and Speak-Out
8/87	Robins/Rorer merger solidified	
10/87		4th newsletter published
11/87	Court hearing on the estimation of the total value of Dalkon Shield claims	Richmond press conference: attack on reorganization plan
12/10/87	Judge sets total value of Dalkon Shield claims at $2.38 billion	
12/17/87	(9 A.M.) Robins announces plan for new merger with a French firm (Sanofi)	(11 A.M.) Press conference at National Press Club: attack reorganization plan

Date	Court Events	DSIN Events
1/19/88	AHP reenters and wins "bidding war," with $2.48 billion for Dalkon Shield claims	
2/3/88	AHP and Robins submit new reorganization plan to the court	
2/6-8/88		Richmond conference: coordinated plan of attack on reorganization plan
3/88		5th newsletter published
3/21/88	Court hearing on adequacy of reorganization plan	DSIN objections to plan presented during court hearing
4/12/88	Five trustees selected to head Dalkon Shield Claimants' Trust	
4/25/88	Ballots for vote on the reorganization plan are mailed to all eligible to vote, includes some 195,000 Dalkon Shield claimants	
5/88		Coalition press conference, urging *no* vote on reorganization plan
7/88	Court hearing to approve merger plan after landslide vote in favor of plan	Hicks removed forcibly from courtroom during approval hearing
8/23/88	Appeal of reorganization plan filed with Fourth Circuit by Public Citizen	
8/25/88	Judge criticizes trustees of Dalkon Shield Claimants' Trust	
9/88	Judge orders investigation of trustees	6th newsletter published
10/88	Court hearing on allegations against trustees	DSIN leaders attend hearing
11/88	Judge fires three trustees	
12/88	Fourth Circuit holds appeals hearing; Trust fund makes first offers of $725	DSIN leaders attend hearing
6/89	Fourth Circuit upholds adequacy and fairness of reorganization plan	DSIN asks Public Citizen not to carry appeal to Supreme Court
9/89	Public Citizen files appeal of reorganization plan to Supreme Court	
11/89	Supreme Court denies appeal	
12/89	AHP concludes buyout of Robins; Dalkon Shield Claimants' Trust receives $2.38 billion in cash	

Appendix C
Letter on Missed Fatherhood

Note: This letter was written by Russell Stone, the husband of Mary Stone (who was rendered sterile by the Dalkon Shield), on the loss of his chance for fatherhood.

May 5, 1988

Dear Son or Daughter,

I write this letter to you because I don't know what else to do. You never existed. You were never born. You never even had a chance to be born because of a mistake your mother and I made a long time ago.

Back in 1970, when your mother and I were married, we had already decided to hold off having children until we felt we could give them the best life possible, so your mother and I agreed together to use a birth control device. We chose the Dalkon Shield IUD. That was a mistake! One that we have both paid for very dearly.

You see, my son or daughter, the Dalkon Shield was a device that was both unsafe and, in some cases, deadly. We didn't know that. The inventor (Dr. Hugh Davis) and the manufacturer (A. H. Robins) did. But they didn't tell anyone! So your mother had it in her body for almost 7 years, thinking it was okay. But it wasn't.

On December 19, 1977, at about 11 P.M., the doctor at the hospital told me and your mom that if he didn't operate right away that night and give your mother a complete hysterectomy, she would die! The infection that the IUD had caused to happen in so many other women had happened in your mom. What could we do? What could your mother do? What could I do? We agreed to the operation.

About four and one-half hours later, the doctor came down the hall (all sweaty and very, very tired) to the waiting room where I was and told me it was done. "Your wife is in recovery," he said. It was done. All your mother's eggs had been removed. She would never have a child or be a mother. I would never be a father. You would never be born.

Sometimes I feel such a hate in my heart because of these people. Sometimes I want to hurt them as much as they hurt us. But what good would that do? You still wouldn't be here. I ask myself: What kind of a world do I live in? That people would hurt other people this way just for money? I get no answer. It is known now, by a lot of people and the supposed justice system, how evil these people are and what they did and then tried in every deceitful way to cover up. Yet still the battle rages to make them pay. At least in a monetary way. But I don't think they really know or believe just how bad they are. And I don't think they'll ever really pay.

But in the meanwhile, you were never born and you are not here. No Little League games. No Sunday outings. No shared plastic model building times. No pretty new dress. No first kiss. No high school. No marriage. No grandchildren. No nothing.

Sometimes at work the other men talk about their kids. About how this one is good in swimming class or that one did something funny in front of everybody. Or how this one is changing jobs. Or that one is good with tools or something. I have to just sit and listen and take it. Sometimes it really hurts, but I just take it.

It's not that I just want a child so I can show him off. If it were only that. I helped raise a couple of brothers so I know what a pain in the butt kids can be sometime. I know there are bad times with kids just like everything else. But sometimes when I hear them talking at work, or I see a baby diaper ad on television or I see a kid walking with their parents, I think of a little pair of arms. A little pair of arms around my neck. A little voice saying DADDY! What I would give for that!

How little those people who have that know. A little pair of arms around my neck and the little voice that says *daddy*.

They say you usually feel better when you get something off your chest. I guess that's what this letter was supposed to do. But I don't feel any better. I feel the same way as when I started . . . empty.

Your father who never was nor will be,

Russell M. Stone

Notes

CHAPTER 1

1. All litigation against Robins was frozen when the company filed for Chapter 11 protection. This included some 9,000 Dalkon Shield lawsuits, a large class-action suit against Aetna (Robins's insurer), and a grand jury investigation of criminal charges, which is a different type of litigation.

2. The Aetna Surety and Casualty Company had insured Robins for many years. Several prominent plaintiff lawyers have amassed substantial documentation of Aetna's complicity with Robins in suppressing information about the injuries and dangers that could have prevented this catastrophe.

3. Robert R. Merhige, Jr., a U.S. District Court judge in Richmond, was assigned to this case the same day Robins petitioned for U.S. Bankruptcy Court protection. Douglas Bragg, an attorney from Denver, attempted to have Judge Merhige recused from this case. The following information is taken from the brief submitted to the court by Bragg: Merhige lives in the same neighborhood and has played golf at the same country club as Mr. Robins for the past 25 years. Judge Merhige's personal attorney coincidentally had represented the Robins Company for many years. Judge Merhige received his law degree at the University of Richmond and is on the law faculty there, where the Robins family is widely acknowledged as its primary benefactor (Bragg, 1986, pp. 118–125). In 1985, the year Robins filed for Chapter 11 protection, the University of Richmond named a new research center the Robert R. Merhige, Jr., Center for Environmental Studies (University of Richmond, 1986). Bragg was unsuccessful in his efforts to have Judge Merhige recused from the case.

CHAPTER 2

1. Such medical abuses are not confined only to women. The asbestos disaster rivals the Dalkon Shield as one of the worst cases of corporate misconduct in producing horrific diseases in men who worked in the asbestos

industry (small numbers of women also worked in this industry and were equally affected).

CHAPTER 3

1. The bankruptcy court was not prepared or equipped to deal with massive numbers of claimants; however, they did not even provide the most basic information, such as the fact that there was a Claimants' Committee to represent them in the court case or that women should begin to gather their medical records immediately. Both of these informational items were of central importance to the legal rights and interests of Dalkon Shield claimants.

2. This woman had authored an early history of the case and had, with several other lawyers, filed motions in 1986 to try to move the bankruptcy proceedings out of Richmond.

3. In the 1970s, Karen Silkwood, a blue-collar worker at the Kerr-McGee power plant, died in a car crash on her way to a meeting with a reporter from the *New York Times*. She was intending to expose what she had discovered about the dangers of plutonium contamination at the plant. The cause of the accident is hotly disputed to this day (Spence, 1989). Her story was dramatized in a Hollywood movie. The Silkwood metaphor for DSIN members was related to the feelings of vulnerability that we had in publicly challenging a major corporation.

4. As I later discovered through experience, the timetable was not unusually slow for this type of court proceeding. In the final analysis, Robins entered Chapter 11 in August 1985 and emerged in December 1989.

5. On the day Robins filed its Chapter 11 petition, it also filed and won motions to keep jurisdiction over the Dalkon Shield issues in the U.S. District Court, rather than turn them over to the U.S. Bankruptcy Court. U.S. District Court Judge Robert R. Merhige, Jr., was appointed to the case on the same day (Schwadel, 1985).

6. During the next year, many lawyers purchased large, regional sections of the list and openly solicited for clients, a controversial practice debated on ethical grounds within the legal profession.

7. Richmond residents were generally well informed about the entire case and issues as a consequence of such thorough news coverage. We received much emotional support and encouragement from Richmond residents we networked with, and we also encountered great anger toward and censure of A. H. Robins. Our original fears about going to Richmond were erased.

8. This is not a trivial strategy. Many reporters will not write a story if they have to do too much background research. Furthermore, our group was quoted correctly because we provided written texts of DSIN speeches in every packet mailed to the press.

9. The most numerous responses always came from the mainstream women's publications (e.g., *Women's World*, a supermarket check-out maga-

zine), and not from publications dealing with issues of social injustice, such as *Ms.* or the *Village Voice*.

10. According to the Bankruptcy Code, a company under Chapter 11 protection must submit its bills to the court and receive court authorization to spend company funds. Robins had given bonuses to its top executives without court authorization, which resulted in the contempt citation.

11. According to U.S. Bankruptcy Code, all *creditors* of a company in Chapter 11 must approve the reorganization plan negotiated by all the committees representing the diverse interest groups. Because the Dalkon Shield claimants were all considered creditors of the company, each one was entitled to vote within their *class* of claims. (Other classes included the company shareholders, the trade creditors, the Internal Revenue Service, the pensioners, the banks, etc.) The Dalkon Shield case and the Johns-Manville (asbestos) cases, in which thousands of injured parties had this right to vote, set precedents in bankruptcy law. However, almost none of the Dalkon Shield claimants understood that they had this right until, at the end of the negotiation process, they received a large (approximately 150-page), legalese-ridden document in the mail, accompanied by a ballot.

Furthermore, historically in bankruptcy cases, the vote is weighted by the relative value of each creditor's shares. In the Dalkon Shield case, however, the judge ruled "one *man*, one vote" (emphasis mine) for all Dalkon Shield creditors, since the individual values of each claim had not been established. This became one of the issues fought (and lost) on appeal. In the end, women would not know the potential value of their individual claims until March 1990, at the earliest. By that time, the trustees of the Dalkon Shield Claimants' Trust would finally have mailed instructions on how to proceed with the review of claims for compensation.

12. I was told later that Judge Merhige could have cited me with contempt of court.

13. In an unusual action, the lawyers for the Claimants' Committee filed an affidavit, alleging questionable conduct by a U.S. district judge. They presented highly specific charges of his unwarranted interference in his insistence that the Trust be located in Richmond, that it employ Richmond people, that it place its money in Richmond banks, and that it give its legal business to Richmond law firms (Mintz, 1988).

CHAPTER 4

1. We returned to the YWCA many times for press conferences and other events during our active protest phase. They welcomed us with open arms, despite the fact that the local United Way, an organization to which Robins contributed heavily, threatened to reduce their funding. We are eternally grateful for their support in the face of institutional and personal risk.

2. Norplant is a subdermal implant, consisting of five match-size cap-

sules, each containing the synthetic progestin levonorgestrel. This hormone is slowly released through the walls of the capules over five years. Depo Provera is an injectable, which contains a long-acting synthetic progesterone. It is usually given as a shot every three months. It was approved for use by the FDA in 1992.

3. In 1992, NWHN affirmed its support for the availability of RU-486 in the United States, but it has at least raised the issue of safety in the *Network News* by offering commentary from experts on both sides of the safety issue (Callum, 1992; Klein, Dumble, & Raymond, 1992). On the other hand, NWHN stated its opposition to FDA approval of Depo Provera as a contraceptive because of grave questions about safety (Neil, 1992). What is the reason for the different postures?

4. Although DSIN was featured widely in many national newspapers and magazines during the first year of its existence, there was no feminist-oriented coverage of this protest movement until the middle of the second year of DSIN's public life.

5. IUDs work partially by preventing implantation of a fertilized egg. Many well-documented Dalkon Shield injuries include septic abortions and ectopic pregnancies.

6. Seven different committees were involved in the Robins bankruptcy: the equity shareholders, the unsecured (trade) creditors, the IRS, the Robins pensioners, the Robins corporation, the Dalkon Shield claimants, and the Dalkon Shield future claimants.

7. Judge Merhige fired the original 38-member Claimants' Committee (mostly plaintiff lawyers with long Dalkon Shield experience) because of the factions that developed among them over whether to cooperate with the bankruptcy proceedings or to continue to fight Robins (Mintz, 1986b). This action came on the heels of a motion by some of those attorneys to seek Merhige's removal from the case (Mintz, 1986b).

8. We resorted to note taking because no one in DSIN could afford to buy official transcripts: Shirley Nichols requested transcripts for just one hearing and was informed that the cost was $4,800.

9. Ann Samani, the former claimant trustee and bankruptcy court administrator in Kentucky, at whom Judge Merhige directed anger for her "open defiance of the court authority," was nominated to a federal judgeship in 1990.

10. The legal specialty that handles cases such as the one involving the Dalkon Shield is called personal-injury law. Such lawyers are trial lawyers, and they bring cases against large institutions, such as airlines, hospitals, doctors, and insurance companies.

11. However, the court did not tell women to gather their medical records, an omission that meant thousands, if not hundreds of thousands, of them would never get the evidence they needed to receive a good settlement. As each year passed, the prospects of securing old medical records diminished. The Trust began publishing its own newsletter in July 1989, a

few months before settlements were to begin. This was the first time officials instructed women to obtain their medical records.

12. DSIN telephone staffers received numerous calls from people saying
that their lawyers had never communicated anything to them about the bankruptcy litigation. In some cases, this included not telling the clients about
their having a vote on the reorganization plan.

13. According to an April 1992 update in the *Claims Resolution Report*
(the Trust's newsletter), "unrepresented" women have received a total of $170
million and "represented" women have received a total of $280 million (of
which approximately $100 million goes to the lawyers) so far. What this
newsletter did not explain is the fact that some 115,000 claimants (probably
all unrepresented) had accepted the lowest offer (Option 1) of $725 or *less*.
The newsletter also reports that only about 7,000 claimants, the vast majority of whom were undoubtedly legally represented, received the highest category of awards that range from $750–$200,000 (Option 3), which probably
accounts for most of the $280 million. Some 13,000 other settled claims prob-
ably fall into the midrange of values to a maximum of $5,000 (Option 2),
with the vast majority of them going to legally unrepresented claimants. As
of that date, the trust reported that it had settled with 135,000 claimants,
out of a grand total of approximately 195,000 claimants (*Claims Resolution
Report*, April 1992, p. 4).

In short, although the U.S. Bankruptcy Court reassured claimants that
lawyers were completely unnecessary, virtually all the women who trusted
that assurance wound up with pitifully small amounts, whereas legally represented claimants generally received larger awards.

CHAPTER 5

1. See Bookman and Morgen (1988) for a spirited debate on the question of gendered political thought, including essentialist theories of women's
special roles and gynocentric ways of thinking and acting.

References

Ackelsberg, M. (1988). Communities, resistance, and women's activism: Some implications for a democratic polity. In A. Bookman & S. Morgen (Eds.), *Women and the politics of empowerment* (pp. 297–313). Philadelphia: Temple University Press.

Acker, D. (1973). Electrocardiogram changes with IUD insertion. *American Journal of Obstetrics and Gynecology, 115,* 458–461.

Allen, C. (1989, November 1). RU-486, the French abortion pill: What is safe? *Wall Street Journal,* p. 6.

Altman, L. (1991, April 15). Study finds doubt on danger arising from use of IUDs. *New York Times,* pp. A1, B6.

Are you a victim of this nasty-looking thing? (1989, April 25). *Women's World,* pp. 4–5.

Bacon, K. (1990, January). U.S. birth control lags. *Wall Street Journal,* pp. B1, B6.

Barrett, P. (1987, August 20). Dalkon claimants are cleared to sue 3 Robins officials. *Wall Street Journal,* p. 29.

Barrett, P. (1988, March 9). For many Dalkon Shield claimants settlement won't end the trauma. *Wall Street Journal,* p. 29.

Blumberg, R., & West, G. (1989, November). *En/gendering social protest: A women-centered perspective.* Paper presented at the meeting of the American Sociological Association, San Francisco.

Bookman, A., & Morgen, S. (1988). *Women and the politics of empowerment.* Philadelphia: Temple University Press.

Bragg, D. (1986, February 19). Petition for writ of mandamus (motion to disqualify). *In re* A. H. Robins Company, 85-01307-R (U.S. Bankruptcy Court, E. D. Virginia).

Breslin, C. (1989, June). Day of reckoning. *Ms.,* pp. 46–52.

Burkman, R. (1981). Association between intrauterine device and pelvic inflammatory disease. *Obstetrics and Gynecology, 57*(3), 269–276.

Callum, J. (1992, September/October). RU-486: A Dialogue: For. *Network News,* pp. 1,4–5.

Carden, M. (1974). *The new feminist movement.* New York: Sage.

Committee on Government Operations. (1973). *Regulation of medical devices (intrauterine contraceptive devices): Hearings before a subcommittee of the committee on government operations, 93rd Congress* (No. 5270-01971). Washington, DC: U.S. Government Printing Office.

Conference Board, Inc. (1987). *Product liability: The corporate response* (Conference Board Report, 893). New York: Author.

Davis, F. (1991). *Moving the mountain: The women's movement in America since 1960*. New York: Simon & Schuster.

Davis, H. (1970). The shield intrauterine device: A superior modern contraceptive. *American Journal of Obstetrics and Gynecology, 106*(3), 455–458.

Despite liability climate, clinicians predict an IUD comeback. (1986, December). *Contraceptive Technology Update, 7*(12), 142–144.

Eagan, A. (1988, July 5). The damage done: The endless saga of the Dalkon Shield. *Village Voice*, pp. 23–30.

Ehrenreich, B., Dowie, M., & Minkin, S. (1979, November). The charge—Gynocide: The accused—The U.S. Government. *Mother Jones*, pp. 56–72.

Ehrenreich, B., & English, D. (1973). *Complaints and disorders: The sexual politics of sickness*. Old Westbury, NY: Feminist Press.

Ehrlich, P. (1968). *The population bomb*. New York: Ballantine.

Eschenbach, D. (1992, June). Earth, motherhood, and the intrauterine device. *Fertility and Sterility, 57*(6), 1177–1179.

Evaluation of intrauterine contraceptive devices. (1967). *Journal of the American Medical Association, 199*, 647.

Experts debate pill switching to combat noncompliance. (1992, October). *Contraceptive Technology Update*, pp. 149–153.

Falls, K. (1989, December). Women's reproductive rights—1989. *DSIN Newsletter* (9), pp. 3–4.

Faludi, S. (1991). *Backlash: The undeclared war against American women*. New York: Crown.

Farley, T., Rosenberg, M., Rowe, P., Chen, J. H., & Meirik, O. (1992, March 28). Intrauterine devices and pelvic inflammatory disease: An international perspective. *Lancet, 339*, 785–88.

Figley, C. (1985). *Trauma and its wake: The study and treatment of post-traumatic stress disorder*. New York: Brunner/Mazel.

Fine, M. (1986). Contextualizing the study of social injustice. In M. Saks & L. Saxe (Eds.), *Advances in applied social psychology* (Vol. 3; pp. 103–126). Hillsdale, NJ: Erlbaum.

Fine, M. (1987). Silencing in public schools. *Language Arts, 64*(2), 157–174.

Fraser, L. (1988, June). Pill politics. *Mother Jones*, pp. 31–33, 44.

Freeman, J. (1975). *The politics of women's liberation: A case study of an emerging social movement and its relation to the policy process*. New York: McKay.

Freire, P. (1970). *Pedagogy of the oppressed*. New York: Continuum.

Freire, P. (1985). *The politics of education: Culture, power, and liberation*. South Hadley, MA: Bergin & Garvey.

Garcia, K. (1989, October 31). 13 women's clinics to be shut by county. *Los Angeles Times*, pp. A1, A22.

Geyelin, M. (1990, January 12). Criminal investigation of A. H. Robins and former law firm is dropped by U.S. *Wall Street Journal*, p. B2.

Gibbs, L. (1992, August). Women warriors. *Everyone's Backyard, 10*(4), 2.

Gilligan, C. (1982). *In a different voice.* Cambridge, MA: Harvard University Press.

Gitlin, T. (1990). Making protest movements newsworthy. In D. Graber, *Media power in politics* (2nd ed.; pp. 276–286). Washington, DC: Congressional Quarterly Press.

Glaberson, W. (1985, October 14). Did Searle close its eyes to a health hazard? *Business Week*, pp. 120–122.

Gladwell, M. (1989, January 22). Lawyers' fees in Dalkon Shield case under fire. *Washington Post*, pp. H8–H9.

Glendinning, C. (1990). *When technology wounds.* New York: Morrow.

Gordon, L. (1977). *Woman's body, woman's right: A social history of birth control in America.* New York: Penguin.

Groups in USA and Europe promote discussion on RU-486. (1989, October). *Women's Global Network for Reproductive Rights*, No. 31, p. 11.

Haire, D. (1984). *How the FDA determines the "safety" of drugs.* (Booklet prepared for the National Women's Health Network, 1325 G St. NW, Washington, DC 20005).

Hardon, A., & Achthoven, L. (1990, November). Norplant: A critical review. *Women and Pharmaceuticals Bulletin*, pp. 14–18.

Hartmann, B. (1987). *Reproductive rights and wrongs.* New York: Harper & Row.

Hartsock, N. (1979). Feminism, power, and change: A theoretical analysis. In B. Cummings & V. Schuck (Eds.), *Women organizing: An anthology* (pp. 2–45). Metuchen, NJ: Scarecrow.

Hatcher, R., Guest, F., Steward, F., Stewart, G., Trussell, J., Cerel, S., & Cates, W. (1986). *Contraceptive technology 1986–1987* (13th rev. ed.). New York: Irvington Publishers.

Health department backs off over Depo-Provera. (1992, March). *Women's Health Watch* [newsletter of the Fertility Action Trust and the Women's Health Information Service, Auckland, New Zealand], p. 2.

Hoen, E. (1990, November). Women and pharmaceuticals: Current concerns. *Women and Pharmaceuticals Bulletin*, pp. 3–8.

Hoffman, M. (1991, October 11). Feminist group dissents on RU-486 use for abortion. *Science, 254*, 199.

Interview with Joseph Mamana. (1973, September 8). *National Observer*, pp. 13–18.

Irishwomen to share in compensation from U.S. IUD maker. (1989, November 18). *Irish Voice*, p. 10.

IUDs may promote infection through design, use of copper. (1987). *Contraceptive Technology Update, 8*(5), 68.

Jacobsen, J. (1983, June). Promoting population stabilization: Incentives for small families. In *Worldwatch Paper 54*. Washington, DC: Worldwatch Institute.

Joreen, A. (1976, April). Trashing: The dark side of sisterhood. *Ms.*, pp. 53–55.

Joseph, A. (1992, November/December). India's population "bomb" explodes over women. *Ms.*, pp. 12–14.

Keith, L., & Berger, G. (1984). The etiology of pelvic inflammatory disease. *Research Frontiers in Fertility Regulation, 3*(1), pp. 1–16.

Kidder, L., & Fine, M. (1986). Making sense of injustice: Social explanations, social action, and the role of the social scientist. In E. Seidman & J. Rappaport (Eds.), *Redefining social problems and reexamining social myths* (pp. 49–63). New York: Plenum.

Kirshon, B., & Poindexter, A. (1988). Contraception: A risk factor for endometriosis. *Obstetrics and Gynecology, 71*(6), 829–831.

Klein, R., Dumble, L., & Raymond, J. (1992, September). RU-486: A dialogue: Against. *Network News*, pp. 1, 6–8.

Kronmal, R., Whitney, C., & Mumford, S. (1991). The intrauterine device and pelvic inflammatory disease: The women's health study reanalyzed. *Journal of Clinical Epidemiology, 44*(2), 109–122.

Labaton, S. (1988a, September 5). Battle for control of Robins case. *New York Times*, p. B28.

Labaton, S. (1988b, July 3). A case to cap a controversial career. *New York Times*, p. F4.

Labaton, S. (1988c, November 29). Judge removes 3 trustees of the Dalkon Shield fund. *New York Times*, pp. D1, D5.

Lang, S. (1988, August). The new IUD: The enemy within? *Vogue*, pp. 230–232.

Lather, P. (1986). Research as praxis. *Harvard Education Review, 56*(3), 257–277.

Lee, N., Rubin, G., Ory, H., & Burkman, R. (1983). Type of intrauterine device and the risk of pelvic inflammatory disease. *Obstetrics & Gynecology, 62*(1), 1–6.

Levine, A. (1982). *Love canal: Science, politics, and people.* Lexington, MA: Lexington Books.

Lichtenstein, R. (1990, April 3). Fewer contraceptive choices exist in U.S. than elsewhere. *Allentown Morning Call*, p. D5.

Lorch, D. (1990, April 24). Protesters on the environment tie up Wall Street. *New York Times*, p. B5.

MacPherson, K. (1986). Feminist praxis in the making: The menopause collective. Unpublished doctoral dissertation, Brandeis University, Waltham, MA. (University Microfilms No. 8617017)

Manchester, R. (1983, April 25). *Citizen's petition for a worldwide recall of the Dalkon Shield IUD.* Submitted to the Food and Drug Administration.

Martin, E. (1987). *The woman in the body.* Boston: Beacon.

McQueen, M. (1989, December 1). Bush administration strongly backs overhaul of U.S. product liability laws. *Wall Street Journal*, p. A6.

Miletich, S. (1989, November 7). Lawyers dispute ethics and fees in Dalkon case. *Seattle Post-Intelligencer*, p. A7.

Miller, J. (1986). *Toward a new psychology of women.* Boston: Beacon.

Millett, K. (1970). *Sexual politics.* New York: Avon.

Mintz, M. (1967). *By prescription only.* Boston: Beacon.

Mintz, M. (1985). *At any cost: Corporate greed, women, and the Dalkon Shield.* New York: Pantheon.

Mintz, M. (1986a, January 5). Lawyer confronts Judge Merhige. *Washington Post*, p. F3.

Mintz, M. (1986b, March 5). Lawyers try to remove judge in Robins case. *Washington Post*, pp. C1–C2.

Mintz, M. (1988, August 9). The selling of an IUD. *Washington Post* (Health Section), pp. 12–16.

Mintz, M. (1989a, October 3). Anatomy of a tragedy. *New York Newsday* (Discovery Section), pp. 1, 3, 5–7.

Mintz, M. (1989b, January 22). During trial, an emphasis on Richmond. *Washington Post*, pp. H1, H8.

Mintz, M. (1989c, September 11). When expediency, not law, prevails. *Legal Times*, pp. 28–33.

Mintz, M. (1991, March). Dangers insurance companies hide. *Trial*, pp. 64–72.

Mokhiber, R. (1989). *Corporate crime and violence.* San Francisco, CA: Sierra Club Books.

Morris, T. (1987a, November 4). Panel says Robins fund would violate bankruptcy laws. *Richmond Times-Dispatch*, p. B1.

Morris, T. (1987b, October 13). Robins president fined $10,000. *Richmond Times-Dispatch*, p. A1.

Morris, T. (1988a, July 19). Claimants approve Robins plan. *Richmond Times-Dispatch*, p. A1.

Morris, T. (1988b, August 26). Irate Merhige may replace Dalkon panel. *Richmond Times-Dispatch*, pp. A1, A10.

Morris, T. (1988c, February 7). Robins' family offer called self-serving. *Richmond Times-Dispatch*, p. B3.

Morris, T. (1988d, September 12). Stakes are high in test of wills between judge and Dalkon trustees. *Richmond Times-Dispatch*, p. A14.

Mumford, S., & Kessel, E. (1992). Was the Dalkon Shield a safe and effective intrauterine device? The conflict between case-control and clinical trial study findings. *Fertility and Sterility*, 56(6), 1151–1176.

Navarro, V. (1976). *Medicine under capitalism.* New York: Prodist.

Neil, K. (1992, September). The Depo-Provera battle. *Network News*, p. 5.

Norsigian, J. (1992). The women's health movement in the United States. *Women's Global Network for Reproductive Rights*, No. 39, pp. 9–12.

Perry, S., & Dawson, J. (1985). *Nightmare: Women and the Dalkon Shield.* New York: Macmillan.

Petchesky, R. (1984). *Abortion and women's choice.* New York: Longman.

Professional fees in A. H. Robins for 1987. (1988, April 15). *Turnarounds and Workouts*, p. 7.

Raymond, J., Klein, R., & Dumble, L. (1991). *RU-486: Misconceptions, myths, and morals.* Cambridge, MA: Institute on Women and Technology.

Roberts, L. (1990, February 23). U.S. lags on birth control development. *Science*, p. 909.

Ruzek, S. (1978). *The women's health movement: Feminist alternatives to medical control*. New York: Praeger.

Schmitt, R. (1989, January 18). Survey questions liability crisis at U.S. companies. *Wall Street Journal*, p. B2.

Schwadel, F. (1985, August 22). Robins files for protection of Chapter 11. *Wall Street Journal*, pp. A3, 10.

Scully, D. (1980). *Men who control women's health: The miseducation of obstetricians-gynecologists*. Boston: Houghton-Mifflin.

Scully, D. (in press). *Men who control women's health: The miseducation of obstetricians-gynecologists* (rev. ed.). New York: Teachers College Press.

Seaman, B. (1969). *The doctors' case against the pill*. New York: Doubleday.

Segal, S. J. (1968). Report of the task force on biologic action. In Advisory Committee on Obstetrics and Gynecology, Food and Drug Administration, *Report on intrauterine devices* (pp. 10–23). Washington, DC: Department of Health, Education, and Welfare.

Shallat, L. (1987, November 27). Local women file suits against manufacturer. *Tico Times* (San José, Costa Rica), p. 5A.

Smith-Rosenberg, C. (1973). Puberty to menopause: The cycle of femininity in nineteenth-century America. *Feminist Studies, 1*, 58–72.

Smith-Rosenberg, C., & Rosenberg, C. (1973). The female animal: Medical and biological views of woman and her role in nineteenth-century America. *Journal of American History, 60*, 332–356.

Sobol, R. (1991) *Bending the law*. Chicago: University of Chicago Press.

Spence, G. (1989). *With justice for none*. New York: Times Books.

Sugarman, S. (1990, May 18). The need to reform personal injury law leaving scientific disputes to scientists. *Science, 248*, 823–827.

Sun, M. (1982). Depo-Provera debate revs up at FDA. *Science, 217*(4558), 429.

Sweet, E. (1988, March). A failed revolution. *Ms.*, pp. 75–79.

Tietze, C. (1967, April). Intrauterine contraception: Recommended procedures for data analysis. *Studies in Family Planning, 18*(Suppl.), 1–6.

Tietze, C., & Lewitt, S. (Eds.). (1962). Intrauterine contraceptive devices. In *Proceedings of the First Conference on the IUCD, April 30–May 1, 1962* (p. 154). New York: Excerpta Medica.

Tudiver, S. (1986). The strength of links: International women's health networks in the 1980s. In K. McDonnell (Ed.), *Adverse effects: Women and the pharmaceutical industry* (pp. 187–214). Penang, Malaysia: International Organization of Consumers Unions.

In re A. H. Robins Company, 85-01307-R (U.S. Bankruptcy Court, E. D. Virginia, 1988). Sixth Amended and Restated Disclosure Statement Pursuant to Section 1125 of the Bankruptcy Code.

University of Richmond. (1986). [University brochure].

Waldholz, M. (1991, April 16). Dalkon Shield trust might use new data to limit some payments. *Wall Street Journal*, p. B2.

Waldholz, M., & Freedman, A. (1987, February 13). American Home withdraws Robins bid, citing risks involved in going forward. *Wall Street Journal*, p. 10.

WHO gives intra-uterine devices clean bill of health. (1987, October 12). [Press release of the World Health Organization Media Service, Geneva, Switzerland.]

Wilson, J. (1973). *Introduction to social movements*. New York: Basic Books.

Wolfsfeld, G. (1990). Collective political action and media strategy: The case of Yamit. In D. Graber (Ed.), *Media power in politics* (2nd ed.; pp. 263–275). Washington, DC: Congressional Quarterly Press.

World Bank. (1984). *World development report 1984*. Oxford, England: Oxford University Press.

Young, S. (1989, June). Is the new IUD for you? *Glamour*, pp. 60–61.

Index

A. H. Robins Company, vii, 1. *See also*
  Dalkon Shield intrauterine device
  acquisition by American Home
    Products (AHP), 7, 10, 67, 70, 116
  bankruptcy petition and reorganiza-
    tion, 6–7, 8–10, 50, 58–59, 65–72,
    90–93, 96–100, 112, 173*n*1, 174*n*4.
    See also Dalkon Shield Claimants'
    Committee; Dalkon Shield
    Claimants Trust
  contempt citation, 65, 175*n*10
  denial of wrongdoing, 6, 8, 16
  disbursements for bankruptcy
    litigation, 9–10
  lawsuits against, 47, 51, 52, 173*n*1
  publicity campaign to notify injured
    parties, 6, 36, 40–42, 50–51, 112
  and rage of claimants, 113, 114–116
  value of shareholders' stock, 10
  withholding of information by, 51,
    163–168
Abortion, 17, 21, 46, 84, 133, 157
  and RU-486, 77, 79–81, 83, 150, 157,
    176*n*3
  septic, 1, 4, 176*n*5
Accountability, of pharmaceuticals
  executives, 159
Achthoven, L., 156
Ackelsberg, M., 110
Acker, D., 24
Ackerman, Joanne, 59, 113, 116, 120, 131
Ackhurst, P., 41
Act-Up, 150
Advertisements
  for Dalkon Shield, 29–33, 34, 35
  for permanent estrogen replacement
    therapy, 161
  and television talk shows, 136–137

Aetna Insurance Company
  immunity from Dalkon Shield-related
    litigation, 7, 10, 173*n*1
  withholding of information by, 51,
    173*n*2
Africa, 41
Akhter, Farida, 46–47
Alan Guttmacher Institute, 83
Allen, C., 83
Altman, L., 47
American College of Obstetrics and
  Gynecology, 80
American Home Products (AHP), 58
  acquisition of A. H. Robins company,
    7, 10, 67, 70, 116
*American Journal of Obstetrics and
  Gynecology,* 5
American Medical Association (AMA), 26
American Pharmaceutical Association, 10
American Trial Lawyers Association, 105
Amniocentesis, 18–19
Anger, of Dalkon Shield claimants, 113,
  114–116
Antibiotics, 4, 28
Australia, 42, 43
Awards, monetary damage, 6, 7, 11, 50,
  177*n*13

Bacon, K., 155
Bangladesh, 46–47
Barrett, Paul, 65, 67, 68, 98, 104
Baye, M. B., 41
Berger, G., 24
Bilateral salpingo-oophorectomy, 19
Birth control. *See* Abortion; Birth control
  pills; High-tech contraception;
  Intrauterine birth control devices
  (IUDs); Population control

About the Author

Karen Hicks is currently Director of the Women's Center and Assistant Professor of Psychology at Albright College in Reading Pennsylvania. She teaches human sexuality, feminist theory, and reproductive rights in the Women's Studies program. She earned her Ph.D. in Human Sexuality Education at the University of Pennsylvania in 1990.